Feed Your Defenses: Using Diet to Strengthen Your Immune System

Table of Content

Introduction

A raging pandemic, an aggressive strain of the flu, even the common cold; illnesses can hit us when we least expect them. But what if we had more control in protecting ourselves? Modern science continues to uncover just how much power our daily habits wield in safeguarding that control tower of health defense - the immune system. Research has now demonstrated that the nutrients we consume impact not just our physical energy, but the vigor by which our bodies battle foreign invaders.

The implications of these discoveries around immunity are profound. What if many stubborn health conditions struggling to be managed by conventional medicine could instead be tackled by biohacking the body's innate healing abilities? By simply making informed adjustments to our diets, might we supercharge our internal defenses to beat back everything from recurring infections to chronic inflammation or even cancer?

This is precisely the promise being revealed. Groundbreaking studies have now charted direct links between disease prevention in humans and certain constituents in common whole foods. From the organosulfur compounds in garlic that can help restrain cancer cell growth to polysaccharides in medicinal fungi that rouse virus-fighting interferons, science is tapping into nature's pharmacy to stimuli our intrinsic resistance. Turns out we may not need fancy pharmaceutical fixes to boost immunity – rather the solution has been right in front of us on our dinner plates this whole time!

Yet with busy, modern lifestyles, putting this knowledge into practice can still remain a challenge. Through a comprehensive, evidence-based approach, *Feed Your Defenses* aims to make nourishing your body's protective systems simple and sustainable. By learning to harness science-backed healing foods and tailor your diet to target critical immune pathways, you'll discover how to unlock your body's latent disease-fighting potential naturally and deliciously. Join us as we explore the next frontier in sustainable wellness – training the mighty forces of immunity that already lie within through strategic, empowering nutrition. Let's begin building your lifelong armory against illness by feeding your body's defenses!

Part I: Understanding Your Immune System

Before strategizing how to bolster our intrinsic defenses against illness, we must first understand exactly what composes this complex, prolific system and how it keeps us well. Expanding comprehension of immune functionality has progressed tremendously over recent decades, yet gaps persist even in conventional medical knowledge. New, paradigm-shifting revelations around immunology continue emerging from progressive scientific inquiry.

For instance, we now recognize that immune competency relies heavily upon synergy with several other physiological systems and processes – notably digestion, metabolism, and the vast ecosystem of our microbiome. Additionally, lifestyle factors from stress management to sleep quality can significantly impact the strength of our protective capacities. As this integrative view of immunity comes into clearer focus, so do nuanced dietary strategies for nourishing whole-body wellness through unique chemical constituents in foods.

By initially surveying core concepts around human immunity along with factors that regulate performance, Part I equips us with vital foundational knowledge to inform strategic nutritional support. We will distill key learnings around the various types of immunological cells, native and adaptive immunity, inflammatory signaling, molecular defense cascades, the essential role of the gut and microbiome, as well as lifestyle influencers like daily rhythms and mental health. Consider this background a primer for comprehending exactly what defense forces comprise your inner healing arsenal, how they function to keep you well, and key areas we will target through targeted, immune-enhancing nutrition.

While delving into the intricacies of immunology may seem daunting at first, grasp of several integral mechanisms will lend invaluable context for the dietary applications to follow. Whether completely new to the workings of immunity or looking to expand your working knowledge, Part I supplies core insights into this profoundly consequential guardian of health – our ever-vigilant immune system.

Chapter 1: An Overview of the Immune System

Imagine an intricate network of specialized cells, tissues, organs, and signaling molecules all orchestrated to protect your health on multiple fronts. Some stand prepared to rapidly respond within minutes against familiar invaders, while others adapt over days to recognize emerging threats never before encountered. Like an elite squadron of microscopic soldiers, the components of this defense force continually surveil all tissues, neutralizing anything that should not be there so that you can go about your day safely.

This remarkable multilayered guardian keeping perpetual watch over your wellbeing is the human immune system – an extraordinarily complex biological defense network that equals the brain in technical sophistication. From venomous spider bites to the common cold, influenza, and pathogens that cause deadly plagues, the immune system tirelessly tackles all biological threats both outside and within. But how exactly does immunity achieve such a monumental feat day after day through an entire human lifetime?

Chief Defense Strategies

Generally speaking, the immune system safeguards your health using two core defense strategies:

Innate immunity involves general protections that kick in immediately against any foreign bodies. These rapidly mobilized responses rely on physical barriers like skin and mucus membranes, defensive immune cells (like macrophages that literally consume pathogens), antimicrobial enzymes, signaling proteins that amplify immune response, and inflammation.

Adaptive immunity develops specialized countermeasures against specific pathogens over days or weeks following exposure. This sophisticated system can establish "immunological memory" as well – meaning once exposed to a threat, adaptive cells like T-lymphocytes and B-lymphocytes retain molecular memories for much faster response upon subsequent encounters with that same intruder.

Immune System Components

The immune system comprises many types of wandering cells circulating in tissues and lymphatic fluid as well as fixed tissues strategically located at potential pathogen entry points. Let's survey some of the key cellular and tissue players involved:

White blood cells like **lymphocytes, monocytes,** and **granulocytes** make up a highly motile cellular workforce detecting threats, communicating alarms to other cells, consuming foreign material through phagocytosis, and coordinating appropriate counteroffensives. Lymphocytes in particular instigate tailored responses to individual pathogens.

Mast cells and **basophils** contain and release inflammatory compounds bringing other immune warriors to problem sites. **Dendritic cells** act like microbial forensic investigators, analyzing foreign material and presenting evidence to adaptive lymphocytes to mount a more specialized response.

The **thymus** and **bone marrow** comprise "training grounds" for maturing T-lymphocytes and B-lymphocytes before deployment into circulation. These primary lymphoid organs equip cells with capacities like self-antigen tolerance to not attack native body tissues.

Secondary lymphoid organs host meet up points for antigen presentation and lymphocyte activation. Key sites include **lymph nodes, tonsils, adenoids, spleen,** and clusters of immune tissue in the small intestine called **Peyer's patches**. Within these locations, innate cells analyze threats and rally adaptive responses from naïve lymphocytes.

Lines of Immune Defense

With various cell types and organs serving specialized roles, investigating immune function can feel overwhelmingly complex. To simplify understanding, we can examine immunity in terms of four escalating lines of defense deployed against any foreign biological material (known as an **antigen** or simply **pathogen**):

1. Physical Barriers

The first line of defense involves simple physical obstructions to keep pathogens completely out of the body. Skin forms an impermeable barrier against most microbes. Similarly, mucus coating respiratory and gastrointestinal tracts traps antigens to be mechanically expelled by coughing or peristaltic movements.

2. Innate Immunity

Should a pathogen circumvent physical barriers, the rapid innate immune response engages. Resident macrophages and mast cells detect foreign material and release signaling proteins called cytokines, unleashing an inflammatory cascade. This summons an army of phagocytic defenders to consume pathogens while natural killer cells assassinate compromised cells.

3. Adaptive Immunity

If innate immunity cannot swiftly neutralize an antigen, the adaptive system develops a custom response over days or weeks tailored to that specific threat. B-lymphocytes mass produce antibodies that mark pathogens for destruction while cytotoxic T-lymphocytes murder infected cells. Memory T and B-cells retain imprints of the antigen to enable future rapid reactions if encountered again.

4. Cell-Mediated Immunity

The most targeted adaptive response against viruses inside cells and cancerous growths is cell-mediated immunity. Cytotoxic T-cells inject infected cells with toxins to destroy both microbe and malignant host cell alike. This constitute the immune system's last line of internal cellular defense before antibodies from humoral (extracellular fluid) immunity.

While additional complexity resides within each stage, this framework provides helpful orientation of how the many immunological pieces mobilize together in sequence to repel disease. Now let's examine some key molecular events underlying immune response.

Signaling Cascades in Immune Activation

Like emergency first responders, immune cells remain dormant until receiving an alarm call. Pathogen detection initiates complex intracellular signaling cascades that activate cellular defenses and genetic transcription of protective compounds.

Pathogen Recognition

Cells identify foreign material via receptors that bind surface proteins or nucleic acids associated with microorganisms but absent in host cells. Toll-like receptors (TLRs) and other pattern recognition receptors (PRRs) detect these unique microbial motifs known as **pathogen-associated molecular patterns (PAMPs)**.

Cell Signaling Pathways

Ligand-receptor binding sets off protein kinase enzyme systems including NF-κB and MAPK that activate downstream gene expression of inflammatory cytokines, antibodies, and antimicrobial peptides while also ramping up core cellular machinery involved in immune processes like phagocytosis.

JAK-STAT pathways subsequently transmit extracellular cytokine signals intracellularly to the nucleus to further modulate gene transcription for immune cells to proliferate and attack pathogens through mechanisms like oxidative bursts.

Cell Death Signaling

When immune cells bind infected cells marked for destruction, molecular interactions trigger signaling proteins (like granzymes) that activate caspase cascades within target cells. These proteolytic enzymes degrade proteins and dismantle the cell from within through regulated cell death (RCD) pathways.

While communication networks involved in immune response can boggle the mind in intricacy, their coordinated signaling enables immune cells to pool information, summon reinforcements, eliminate threats, clean up collateral damage, and return to homeostasis.

Now that we have reviewed some foundational concepts around our elaborate immunological defense systems, subsequent chapters will uncover how other bodily processes intimately tied to immune health wield equal or greater influence. This interdependent, holistic perspective of human immunity forms the basis for many nutrition-based biohacking strategies – identifying ideal therapeutic food compounds that can simultaneously nourish multiple bodily systems underlying disease resistance and vital longevity.

Chapter 2: Gut Health and Immunity

While most might assume the immune system operates independently, new revelations demonstrate that several other major physiological processes share an intimate, inseparable connection with defensive competency. Chief among them is the digestive system – or more specifically, the vast microbiome inhabiting our gastrointestinal tract. These trillions of microbes powerfully shape immune cell development, education, regulation, and nearly all facets of both innate and adaptive responses. Misguided health notions of "boosting immunity" independent of the gut do little to impact holistic disease resilience. To biohack robust protection, we must first feed the pillars of total immune integrity: the gut and its microbiome.

Gut Immunity Starts Early

Even before birth, certain gut microbes prompt immune tissue development. During gestation, a tolerant "instructor" class of Clostridia species establishes a healthy scaffolding of skin and intestinal barriers, regulatory cells, cytokine balance, IgA antibodies, Toll-like receptors, and lymph nodes shortly after the first trimester. Disrupting this fetal process may help explain modern epidemics of allergies, asthma, eczema and autoimmunity.

Like distribution networks carrying resources across territory, gut microbes forge infrastructure that immune and metabolic traffic depends upon. Babies born via cesarean lack healthy seed microbes acquired from natural vaginal childbirth. This deficiency can predispose immune abnormalities like allergies and asthma later in life. Consequently, mimicking vaginal birth exposure through gently swabbing an infant's newly exposed skin and mouth with the mother's vaginal microbes can prevent immune dysfunction.

Clearly from our earliest days, friendly microbes guide the balanced molding of lifelong immunological health.

GALT: Where Immunity Meets Microbiome

Where exactly in physiology do this cooperative convergence between host immunity and microbes occur? Our intestinal tract houses a vast network of immune organs and tissues interfacing the rich inner and outer microbial worlds.

Gut-Associated Lymphoid Tissue (GALT) constitutes the largest immune compartment comprising 70% of all our body's defenses. An expansive surface area exceeding 40 square meters provides prime real estate for vital crosstalk between 100 trillion bacteria and the intestinal immune system.

Here hundreds of lymph nodes, antibody-activated immune cells in Peyer's patches, rows of immunosurveillance microfold (M) intestinal cells, isolated lymphoid follicles, and large armies of roaming dendritic cells, macrophages, mast cells and innate lymphoid cells (ILCs) continually sample gut contents. These flat villi structures allow nutrients to pass efficiently while filtering toxins and pathogens.

Like a bustling harbor receiving ships and commodities from afar, the portals of intestinal villi enable thriving commerce between host mitochondria and foreign molecular imports ferried by diverse microbiota. This heavy traffic feeds and regulates local immune dialogue that echoes systemically, impacting holistic wellness far beyond mere digestion.

Mucosal Barrier Integrity

This extensive surveillance network relies on intact tight junctions sealing epithelial barriers between villi to operate properly. Disrupted intestinal lining – clinically referred to as "leaky gut" – fosters inflammation that can trigger wide-ranging immune dysregulation manifesting as food sensitivities, allergies, and autoimmunity.

Many lifestyle factors like chronic stress, sleep deprivation, alcohol consumption, NSAID pain relievers and nutrient-poor diets high in saturated fats and refined carbohydrates destabilize mucosal integrity. Alternatively, compounds like glutamine, vitamin A, zinc and polyphenols reinforce tight junctions.

Assessing blood markers like lipopolysaccharide, zonulin and intestinal fatty acid binding protein help identify impaired barriers requiring structural nutrition and microbiome restoration before adverse downstream immune consequences arise.

Microbiome Mapping Advances Immune Insights

Beyond bolstering borders, care of our internal microbial community directly steers host immune capability as well. Sophisticated gene sequencing platforms now enable accurate mapping of human microbiome inhabitants to gauge community diversity and functional capacities. Comparing healthy and diseased states reveals influential microbe tribes that shape inflammatory dynamics.

Research groups like the Integrative Human Microbiome Project (HMP) report only a small percentage differ between individuals. Core symbionts like Faecalibacterium prausnitzii hold valuable anti-inflammatory properties and remain depleted among autoimmune conditions. Such common deficiencies provide target species to augment through diet for favorable immunomodulation.

Ongoing microbiome analytics continues illuminating key members that drive immune outcomes. For instance, a shortfall in normally protective Bifidobacteria induces worsened influenza outcomes in mice by limiting antiviral interferon-λ production from lung epithelial cells during infection. Incredible power may reside in recolonizing such depleted yet vital species.

Microbial Imprinting Educates Immunity

Beyond bolstering borders and mapping influencers, gut flora play an even more direct role shaping host immunity: immune education through "training" leukocytes about what compounds to attack or tolerate. This process begins with unique sugars coating microbial membranes that mirror similar carbohydrate patterns found on foods and human tissues.

Dendritic immune cells sample intestinal bacteria and migrate to mesenteric lymph nodes where they "present" these membrane sugars to naive T-cells, teaching them not to overreact to identical carbohydrate patterns on gluten, birch pollen or joint cartilage. Mistakes in this chemical identification education early in life fosters hypersensitivity disorders like celiac disease or rheumatoid arthritis.

Consuming fermented foods like yogurt and kefir containing polysaccharide-enrobed microbes or metabolizing complex carbs from whole plant foods into short-chain fatty acids both help guide proper immune imprinting for lasting food tolerance and tempered reactions.

Microbiota Influence Immune Development

Beyond basic tolerance schooling, gut flora actively shape distribution, availability and maturation of various leukocytes. Germ-free mice display abnormal immune cell counts and activity compared to conventional mice. Their off-kilter portfolio includes fewer B and T-lymphocyte reserves, excessive dendritic and natural killer cells, reduced macrophage phagocytic efficiency, dysbiotic cytokine signaling, perpetual systemic inflammation with eosinophilia and compromised secondary lymphoid organs.

Recolonizing the deficient microbiome normalizes these aberrant immune manifestations. Additionally, adolescence marks a window where microbiome flux drives maturation of adult regulatory and TH17 intestinal lymphocytes for strengthened mucosal immunity. Disrupted community patterns during this critical juncture also raise later life autoimmune risks.

Clearly gut microbes direct both prenatal developmental pathways and postnatal adaptive education essential for future balanced immunity. Their intimate body partnership places commensal bacteria equally alongside our human genome in governing lifelong health expression.

Short-Chain Fatty Acids Regulate Immunity

Microbes further shape host defenses through their major digestive byproduct – short-chain fatty acids (SCFAs). Fermenting otherwise indigestible fibers from whole plant foods, gut bugs transform complex carbohydrates into bioactive compounds like butyrate, propionate and acetate that integrate metabolism, epigenetics and intestinal homeostasis.

Butyrate concentrates heavily within intestinal cells as their preferred energy substrate, enhancing mucosal integrity while also inhibiting inflammatory NF-kB and NLRP3 pathways via epigenetic histone modification. This fosters epithelial tolerance and homeostasis. Propionate feeds liver gluconeogenesis while acetate bolsters lipid metabolism.

Beyond intestinal health, SCFAs enter circulation signaling through G-protein receptors to reduce neutrophil migration and demonstrate broad anti-inflammatory, antioxidative, tumor-suppressive, insulin-sensitizing, gut barrier-protective and appetite-regulating activities. Clearly these microbial metabolites act as potent immunomodulatory agents with systemic benefits.

Probiotics Show Promise

If specific bacteria so critically shape host immunity, selectively introducing health-promoting species as probiotic supplements holds understandable appeal. Global probiotic sales now exceed $40 billion annually. But with such a bountiful and biodiverse microbiome, can simply up-regulating a few strains realistically enhance holistic health from Alzheimer's disease to depression?

While research continues working to isolate most efficacious species, strains and dosages for precise medical applications, some promising prospects have emerged:

- **Immune resilience** against pathogens improves with Lactobacillus casei supplementation during cold/flu season.

- Multiple probiotic strains reduce **gut inflammation** and reinforce epithelial integrity for **food tolerance** in irritable bowel syndrome.

- Certain Bifidobacterium strains show **antiviral** effects against hepatitis B, influenza virus and norovirus while Lactobacillus rhamnosus increases macrophage activity against bacterial infections like listeria and salmonella.

- In **allergy**, certain lactobacilli reduce symptomatic histamine release and IgE sensitization while protecting airway tissue in asthmatic mice.

- For **autoimmunity**, Lactobacillus casei attenuates development of diabetes in preclinical models by balancing inflammatory T cells and regulatory Tregs. Bifidobacterium infantis alleviates intestinal inflammation in ulcerative colitis patients.

While still an emerging field, select probiotic species clearly hold immunomodulatory significance in certain scenarios. Yet an isolated approach of singular strains fails to address underlying dysbiosis driving most conditions. Improving native microbial richness through dietary fiber diversity and fermented foods offering a spectrum of symbionts will likely better support holistic microbiome-immune dialogue vital for systemic vitality.

Chapter 3: Lifestyle Factors That Impact Immune Function

While equipped with an impressive arsenal of cellular weaponry and molecular defenses, the formidable immune system does not operate in isolation. Far from an autonomous process, immunity relies intimately on multiple bodily systems working synergistically to express optimal performance. Consequently, supporting pillars of total body health simultaneously bolsters disease resistance capacity.

Conversely, lifestyle factors that disturb homeostasis across physiological networks conversely impair immune competence. Chronic inflammation, metabolic disorders, circadian disruption, gut permeability, psychological stress and microbiome imbalance all limit immune resilience.

Fortunately, evidence confirms that adopting practices and consuming compounds that reduce systemic inflammation, improve metabolic flexibility, support detoxification, enable restful sleep, cultivate phytonutrients and probiotics, and process emotional stress can considerably strengthen immune defenses against invading threats.

Inflammation and Immune Activation

As outlined in earlier chapters, acute inflammatory response marks a normal phase of controlled immune activation that eliminates pathogens and initiates tissue healing. However, left unchecked from either pathogenic factors or collateral damage, inflammation can become relentless and self-perpetuating. This smoldering low-grade variety called **chronic inflammation** underlies practically all chronic diseases from dementia to diabetes, cancer to cardiovascular disease.

Intestinal permeability, obesity, sedentary lifestyle, smoking, pollutant exposures and psychosocial stress all feed systemic inflammation that disturbs immune balance by constantly triggering damage signals, even without actual threats present. This false alarm state saps resources by demanding continual immune response and tissue repair while also fostering excessive clotting, aggravated free radical injury, internal autoimmunity against host proteins, and uncontrolled cellular proliferation.

Dampening inflammation and resolving inflammatory signaling pathways therefor holds monumental relevance for both optimizing daily immune function as well as reversing advanced chronic inflammatory conditions.

Immune Health Relies on Metabolic Flexibility

One core tenet of functional nutrition involves appreciation that immune cells rely as much on healthy energy metabolism for peak performance as the brain, muscles or heart. However in modern times with abundant yet often poor quality dietary macronutrients, immune cells frequently battle threats in the context of systemic metabolic dysfunction.

Perpetual high blood sugar, insulin resistance, adipocyte dysfunction with fatty acid excess, mitochondrial oxidative stress and malnourished cellular environments all constrain immunosurveillance capabilities against pathogens and malignant transformations. On the other hand, occasional short-term fasting, exercise, sauna therapy and consumption of anti-inflammatory, antioxidant, polyphenol-rich whole foods all support metabolic health through pathways that bolster immune cells simultaneously.

This interdependent relationship between metabolism and immunity means that conditions like obesity, cardiovascular disease and type 2 diabetes centrally driven by metabolic dysfunction also limit disease resistance precisely when increased immune competence becomes needed most.

By improving glycemic variability, supporting mitochondrial respiration, reducing adipose inflammation, and cultivating metabolic flexibility, the immune cells, organs and signaling networks central to fighting illness receive the substrates, oxygen and molecular messaging to function reliably when threats emerge.

Circadian Biology Influences Immune Rhythms

Our immune defenses adhere to natural circadian fluctuations tuned to cycles of activity, feeding, restfulness and cellular repair across 24 hours. Diurnal oscillations characterize numbers and responsiveness of varied circulating lymphocytes. Cellular machinery involved in DNA repair, apoptosis, digestion/absorption and xenobiotic detoxification all follow comparable rhythmic patterns throughout bodily tissues.

With deep evolutionary roots, these biological timers likely help marshal resources to anticipate changing needs across sleep/wake phases. Supporting healthy regulation of these innate rhythmic immune cycles therefor holds relevance for ensuring cells remain optimally prepared for threats likely to appear at characteristic times of day.

For example, past sunset when feeding ceases, gut macrophages and lymphocytes peak while neutrophils and various blood cell levels dip until dawn when activity resumes. During sleep cycles, worn cellular components undergo lysosomal digestion and recycling in rhythm with metabolic rate fluctuations.

Disrupting homeostatic biological tempo through altered sleep routines or feeding times taxes physiological synchrony required for maximal performance. Night shift work, inconsistent bedtimes, sleep deprivation, circadian gene mutations and exposure to artificial light after dusk all demonstrate immune consequences such as worsened viral infection severity, delayed wound repair, chronic inflammation, tumor progression, metabolic disorders and mood imbalance through disturbed circadian biology.

Fortifying natural light/dark transitions, avoiding food past dusk, enabling restorative sleep, managing technology exposure and properly orchestrating fasting/feeding cycles all help harmonize innate immune rhythms for heightening daily vitality and nighttime repair processes.

Psychological Stress Weakens Immunity

Beyond concrete physiological variables, more ethereal yet equally influential factors like emotional state and perceived life stress also significantly sway immune capability given extensive crosstalk between the endocrine, nervous and immune systems. Inherent survival responses prepare the body for perceived threats including vigilance against infection risks that might increase after experiencing traumatic stress.

By triggering sympathetic nervous system arousal and subsequent hypothalamic release of corticotropin releasing hormone (CRH), adrenocorticotropic hormone (ACTH) and glucocorticoids, the hormonal products released during acute anxiety and distress directly signal immune cells expressing respective receptors. Glucocorticoids like cortisol shut down protective inflammation through immunosuppressive actions.

Elevated baseline levels of CRH, ACTH and cortisol from recurring emotional stress cause relentless immunosuppression, reducing quantities, responsiveness and cytotoxicity of natural killer cells along with suppressed antibody production. These cellular deficiencies then manifest as impaired viral defense plus higher risk for recurring infections and cancer.

While momentary flight-fight reactions can safely contain potential threats, resolution through parasympathetic relaxation nourishes the overturned homeostasis vital for balanced immune potential. Supporting healthy neuroendocrine regulation through stress resilience practices like mindfulness meditation and yoga have shown consistent immunological benefits – decreased inflammatory signaling, improved vaccination response, quicker wound repair, slowed tumor growth and enhanced antiviral defenses resulting in fewer cold/flu symptoms compared to non-adherents. Clearly immunity and emotions remain unavoidably interconnected at foundational levels.

Part II: Foods That Strengthen Immune Defenses

Armed with expanded insight into the countless cellular and molecular interactions comprising our elaborate immune defenses, we now shift focus to discovering how everyday foods can help equip these intricate systems for optimal performance.

While the prospect of bolstering disease resistance through strategic nutrition may sound too good to be true, thousands of contemporary scientific studies now reinforce certain edible plants and their chemical derivatives as profoundly influencing human immune competence.

Of course simply adopting random so-called "immune boosting" supplements likely confers little real-world benefit given the endogenous complexity within physiology. But selectively applying evidence-based functional foods and phytochemicals matched to targeted immune pathways holds genuine promise for supporting this most vital process underlying resilience.

Through the following sections, we will methodically survey key food categories containing compounds shown to beneficially interact with critical defensive functions involved in pathogen identification, inflammatory signaling, microbial imprinting, intracellular antioxidant capacity, DNA protection and repair, apoptosis, digestive permeability, leukocyte proliferation and cytotoxic targeting.

These healing foods provide the raw materials to fuel processes our intrinsic immunological machinery requires for keeping latent threats in check day to day in addition to mounting formidable counteroffensives when invasive agents circumvent initial barriers. Consider each chapter a guide for understanding disease-fighting culinary tools you likely already have easy access to.

While individual needs and health conditions vary, focusing daily nourishment around incorporating more of these immune-supporting edible compounds into balanced menus can strengthen systemic surveillance and response kinetics against opportunistic bacteria, viruses, malignant transformations as well as expedite healing processes – helping you spend less time sick and more time thriving across your lifespan. Let's discover what's on the menu for feeding your formidable defenses!

Chapter 4: Colorful Fruits and Vegetables

While limited nutrients alone cannot wield miracle cures, scientists now widely accept that certain beneficial compounds concentrated in whole plant foods hold capacity to help vital physiology - including our elaborate immune defenses - operate closer to theoretical peak efficiency.

Triggering profound downstream wellness benefits, subtle influences like improving white blood cell membranous fluidity to heighten motility or increasing lysosomal enzymatic recycling capacity of aging neutrophils and macrophages during routine clean-up processes can make the difference in effectively eradicating emerging infections before symptoms fully manifest.

Many divination traditions from Chinese medicine to indigenous African bush lore uphold colorful fruits and vegetables as bestowing heightened vital "life force" - an intuitive concept remarkably validated by contemporary nutritional immunology uncovering specific bioactive chemicals that do seem to literally enhance energetic immunity dynamics.

Responsible for vivid yellow, orange, red, purple, blue, and green hues that attract seed-dispersing animals, phytochemical pigments serve plants not unlike immune cells patrol human tissues - recognizing microbial or invasive threats then neutralizing through phagocytosis while signaling reparative mechanisms. These analogous anti-pathogen properties pass on to us as well.

While all whole produce generally nurtures wellness, the following pigmented varieties offer targeted nourishment to critical processes underlying immune competence:

Carotenoid-Rich: Yellow/Orange Plant Foods

Bananas, pumpkin, sweet potato, carrots, oranges and mangos all house a spectrum of disease-fighting carotenoid compounds such as beta carotene, alpha carotene, beta cryptoxanthin, zeaxanthin and lutein.

These antioxidant phytochemicals concentrate within skin and mucosal membranes enhancing integrity against invasive microbes while also increasing proliferation of macrophages and natural killer cells to ramp up cellular immunity against colon, lung and skin cancers.

Carotenoids further concentrate within immune cells, protecting DNA from free radical damage that can hamper replication and intracellular communication abilities. They likewise aid phagocytic activity helping macrophages and neutrophils effectively consume and destroy engulfed threats.

Select carotenoids convert into usable vitamin A - a micronutrient deficiency notoriously underlying weakened immunity across developing countries. Beyond bolstering epithelial barriers and night vision, vitamin A signals genes that code for bactericidal proteins while also enhancing lymphocyte responsiveness, antibody production, and apoptosis of worn antigen-fighting immune cells.

Ongoing research continues elaborating how versatile carotenoid compounds flexibly tune myriad processes granting immune cells heightened responsivity against numerous pathogenic factors.

Anthocyanin-Rich: Red/Blue Plant Foods

Anthocyanins imparting beautiful red, purple and blue shades signal antioxidant richness in nutrient-dense berries, eggplant skins, black rice, red/purple sweet potatoes, dark grapes and plums.

As flavonoid polyphenol compounds, they quench excessive inflammatory cascades through cytokine modulation and signaling regulation to prevent unchecked immunological damage. Anthocyanins likewise concentrate within cell nuclei enhancing structural integrity of DNA strands inside lymphocytes while improving accurate repair of inevitable errors arising during rapid proliferative cycles.

Tart cherries hold especially valuable anti-gout properties by lowering inflammatory uric acid accumulation. Beyond neutralizing free radicals, red/blue plant anthocyanins assist apoptosis and immune cell turnover for more responsive defenses. They also restrict blood supply to tumors thus slowing mutation proliferation.

Explaining their almost universal presence among global indigenous cuisines, ongoing research continues substantiating how anthocyanin bioactives confer broad-spectrum support through numerous channels that collectively bolster immune resilience.

Allicin-Rich: Pungent Culinary Herbs

Beyond produce, aromatic herbs and spices also amply provide key immune-enhancing phytochemicals, most notably: allicin.

Garlic, onions, leeks and shallots all contain precursors to active allicin - liberated upon crushing cells during chopping or chewing to yield potent sulfur-rich compounds that concentrate near mucus membranes.

Historically used to prevent wound infection before antibiotics, allicin disrupts microbial enzymatic function and cell membranes through oxidation while also suppressing viruses, fungi and intestinal parasites. Further immune benefits include enhancing natural killer cell activity against malignant cells, regulating inflammatory prostaglandins via COX-2 inhibition, chelating heavy metals and underscoring cardiovascular benefits of Mediterranean-style diets.

Taken regularly, aged garlic extract significantly reduces cold and flu severity while clinical indications suggest supplemental aged garlic and antimicrobial herbs like andrographis, elderberry, cinnamon and echinacea help shorten duration of upper respiratory infections in certain individuals.

Yet for everyday resilience, creatively incorporating allicin-releasing foods like crushed garlic, scallions, chives and onions into main dishes and marinades provides continual support against exogenous threats and endogenous aberrant cell growth - helping explain lower cancer rates among those eating ample allium family vegetables.

Glucosinolate-Rich: Cruciferous Vegetables

Another category of sulfur-bearing plant compounds called glucosinolates abundant within cruciferous vegetables like broccoli, kale, arugula, Brussels sprouts, bok choy, cauliflower, collards, cabbage, watercress and horseradish incite similar cytoprotective effects like allicin.

Chewing or chopping ruptures plant cell walls, allowing intrinsic myrosinase enzymes to convert glucosinolates into bioactive isothiocyanates and indole derivatives. Beyond benefiting estrogen metabolism for cancer prevention, these spicy phytochemicals concentrate near mucus membranes enhancing chemical defenses and microcirculation.

They likewise up-regulate endogenous antioxidant capacity while modulating xenobiotic detoxification enzymes for versatile protection across tissue types against many threats. Animal models and cell culture assays demonstrate direct antimicrobial effects with certain bacterial strains in addition to anti-parasitic, antifungal and antiviral influences.

Indole glucosinolates in watercress and arugula specifically limit a cell surface protein that enables carcinogenic HPV to inactivate tumor suppressing p53 proteins inside infected cervical epithelial cells - effectively blocking early cancerous transformations by this prevalent sexually transmitted virus.

Sufficient regular intake alongside allicin-releasing alliums assists the formidable frontline defenses freeze, fight and flush a range of menacing microbes and malignant influences before they jeopardize resilience.

Polyphenol-Rich: Colorful Whole Plant Foods

Finally we arrive at the largest ubiquitous family of defensive plant bioactives: polyphenols. These antioxidant phenolic ring compounds bathe practically all fruits and vegetables to discourage pests, infections and solar damage.

Concentrating in skins, seeds and stems, over 10,000 identified polyphenols like quercetin, catechins, ellagitannins and resveratrol frequently enter studies correlating high produce intake with lowered inflammatory conditions.

Beyond conferring pigments, polyphenols regulate gene expression of cytoprotective proteins, bolster endogenous antioxidants like glutathione, stabilize watchman tumor suppressor p53 activity, influence cell signaling cascades and epigenetics, chelate troublesome iron and copper ions, inhibit microbial efflux pumps and quench nitrogen species that perpetuate chronic inflammation underlying immunosenescence.

Polyphenol bioavailability depends greatly on intestinal microflora that liberate metabolites which then circulate systemically through blood and lymph acting upon tissues. These microbiome-derived phenolic derivatives like hydroxybenzoic acid often convey more potent benefits than their parent compounds. This synergy underscores the importance of fostering microbiome diversity through continual rainbow diets rich in a variety whole plant foods beyond just isolated juices or supplements.

On the whole real, fresh, vibrantly pigmented fruits and vegetables that appease all senses provide a foundational immunological bedrock upon which supplemental targeted phytochemicals can build localized enhancements to shore up daily disease resilience.

Chapter 5: Herbs, Spices, and Teas

Beyond fruits and vegetables, aromatic culinary herbs, spices and traditional medicinal plant infusions provide concentrated sources of bioactive metabolites shown to beneficially interact with human immune cells and signaling cascades.

Complex botanical preparations often outperform isolated constituents by synergistically buffering absorption rates for more sustained potency through dynamic secondary interactions between numerous phytochemicals. Once absorbed, these small xenobiotic molecules readily penetrate immune cell membranes to variously exert antioxidant, anti-inflammatory, antimicrobial and immunomodulatory influences.

While definitive human evidence remains limited on many traditional herbs and spices, rapid expansion of in vitro assays and animal models consistently demonstrate plausible multi-pronged mechanisms by which numerous plant compounds logically combat infectious and inflammatory threats.

As both protective shield and treatment, time-tested herbal tonics and familiar culinary spices present safe, accessible means to optimize daily immune function while managing active symptoms when innate defenses prove overwhelmed. Let's survey some of most promising botanicals for bolstering immunity through targeted support of myriad physiological processes.

Potent Antiviral Herbs

Elderberry, licorice, oregano, garlic, echinacea, astragalus, holy basil, pelargonium sidoides and andrographis all demonstrate antiviral properties against respiratory viruses like influenza, rhinovirus and respiratory syncytial virus (RSV). Further antiviral benefits have been shown against viral hepatitis, HIV, herpes simplex, dengue and varicella zoster.

Derived components like anthrocyanins, glycyrrhizin, carvacrol, allicin, alkylamides, polysaccharides, ursolic acid, aucubin and andrographolide concentrate within lysosomes, cell surface membranes and nuclei of infected immune cells to prevent viral docking, fusion, replication and cytokine storm overreaction through multitude intracellular mechanisms.

These traditional antiviral botanicals used for centuries across Asia, Europe and Americas confirm modern pharmacological relevance both preventing and alleviating severity of viral infections - particularly for influenza prevention and therapy. However quality, processing methods and sourcing all significantly impact clinical effectiveness. Drinking elderberry tea combines cardiovascular polyphenols with antiviral anthocyanins for example. Further human trials aim to validate most efficacious preparations, combinations and therapeutic dosing.

Anti-Inflammatory Herbs

Curcumin, ginger, turmeric, green tea, rosemary, holy basil, garlic, boswellia, thyme, oregano, resveratrol and many medicinal mushrooms demonstrate anti-inflammatory actions beneficial for reducing allergy, autoimmunity, digestive permeability, joint pain, recovery from intense exertion and alleviating chronic inflammatory conditions.

Via modulation of regulatory T cells, suppressing inflammatory cytokines like IL-6, IL-1beta, IL-8 and TNF-alpha, inhibiting COX/LOX enzymes, chelating inflammatory minerals and stabilizing mitochondria against destructive oxidative stress, these potent anti-inflammatory herbs counteract unrestrained inflammatory signaling both acutely and chronically for systemic homeostasis.

Through suppression of specific upstream inflammatory signals, certain extracts effectively treat gastrointestinal conditions like ulcerative colitis, metabolic disorders like fatty liver and vascular conditions like atherosclerosis rooted in uncontrolled inflammation. Their downstream mechanisms likely hold relevance for prevention and therapy of all inflammation-driven immune imbalances.

Immunomodulatory Herbs & Mushrooms

Beyond rigidly boosting or suppressing inflammation, certain botanicals exhibit more nuanced bidirectional immunomodulatory effects - upregulating host defenses against microbial invasion while concurrently attenuating excessive inflammation or isolated overreactive elements.

Species like astragalus, garlic, ginseng, guduchi, cordyceps, turkey tail and reishi mushrooms all enhance macrophage phagocytosis, NK cell toxicity, antigen-specific lymphocyte proliferation and beneficial anti-cancer cytokines like IL-2 and TNF-alpha while rebalancing excessive pro-inflammatory Th2 cytokines.

These intelligent mushrooms and herbs essentially tune and optimize endogenous immune response kinetics for more effective initial threat clearance with minimized unnecessary bystander damage rather than simplistically pushing isolated aspects higher or lower. Further antioxidant, antiviral and nerve-regenerative properties synergize for whole-body upregulation uniquely lacking in pharmaceutical immune suppressants.

Immunoprotective Polyphenol Teas

Common teas derived from antioxidant-rich camellia sinensis leaves additionally exhibit multifaceted upstream immune benefits rooted in polyphenolic compounds like epigallocatechin gallate (EGCG) that concentrate near mucosal membranes.

Green and black teas promote beneficial T regulatory lymphocytes that induce immune tolerance to harmless non-self compounds for prevention of seasonal allergy and autoimmunity. Particular catechins also guard mitochondrial DNA from damage incurred during regular metabolism and oxidant threats that over time can undermine cellular immunity.

Further antibacterial properties against certain oral and intestinal pathogens plus antiviral activity against hepatitis B and influenza along with vascular and metabolic benefits collectively support sustained immune integrity over the lifespan. Many herbal teas offer similar polyphenol-derived resilience.

As vehicles for phytochemicals that interface host physiology through digestion, herbs and spices present versatile methods to beneficially nourish immune cell bioenergetics, signaling proteins and gene transcription factors for daily optimization and acute support when inflammatory symptoms manifest from intrinsic pathogenic weaknesses or extrinsic threats that exploit individual predispositions.

Chapter 6: Fermented Foods and Prebiotics

Beyond direct immune cell interactions, certain functional foods indirectly stimulate defenses by nourishing the vast intestinal microbiome introduced earlier as director of lifelong immune development, education and balanced homeostasis.

By combatting dysbiosis, enhancing native diversity and recolonizing keystone commensals, live-culture fermented foods, fiber-rich prebiotic plant material and possibly select probiotic supplements calibrate microbiome:immune crosstalk for systemic resilience against inflammatory diseases.

Let's examine the immune benefits associated with providing our microbiome hand-selected beneficial microbes and their preferred metabolic substrates.

Fermented Foods - Live Microbial Nourishment

Classically prepared yogurt, kefir, kimchi, sauerkraut, kombucha, miso, tempeh, pickled vegetables and aged cheeses all contain bioactive genera that tangibly interact with human immunity. Beyond basic nutrition, compounds secreted by lactic acid bacteria, acetogenic bacteria and yeast during fermentation uphold diverse benefits.

As native human commensals, fermentative Firmicutes including Lactobacillus, Lactococcus, Enterococcus, Streptococcus, Pediococcus and Leuconostoc species provide immune cells continual training on harmless compounds to ignore compared to foreign antigens requiring active response. Their tasty habitats conveniently supply live "training modulators."

With systemic absorption, some strains reduce inflammatory signaling, reinforce epithelial junctions preventing allergen flux and pathogen invasion, chelate heavy metals, direct tryptophan metabolism away from anxiety-provoking kynurenine, produce neurotransmitters like GABA that suppress pain signaling and modulate anti-cancer lymphocytes - acting as edible probiotics.

As genus complexity matters enormously, traditionally cultured foods likely confer advantages over commercial probiotic capsules by better approximating native niche diversity. Nonetheless, clinical applications for isolated strains hold logic, especially replacing specific commensals like Lactobacillus johnsonii that normally metabolize tryptophan into serotonin yet diminish among those suffering major depression.

Either way, ingesting copious communities of immune-training, inflammation-resolving, antimicrobial, neuroprotective lactic acid microbes through minimally-processed fermented fare provides a strong foundation upon which supplemental species can build localized enhancements like urogenital vaginosis treatment.

Prebiotic Plant Fibers- Feeding Beneficial Microbes

In addition to providing live microbes, certain dietary fibers selectively nourish protective resident organisms like Faecalibacterium prausnitzii that starve without adequate polysaccharides. Called prebiotics, vegetables, fruits and whole grains rich in inulin, fructooligosaccharides, resistant starch, arabinoxylan and other plant cell wall fibers pass undigested into the colon where hungry symbionts awaiting them liberate anti-inflammatory metabolites like butyrate.

By suppressing intestinal permeability and systemic lipopolysaccharide burden alongside heightened SCFA production, prebiotic fiber feeds mechanisms underlying immune balance- promoting diversity through species like Bifidobacterium that possess their own enzymatic toolboxes to unlock energy bound within resilient starch and inulin.

Additional components like polyphenols and minerals further support microbial and immune cell health. Enthusiasm for novel prebiotic supplements like galactooligosaccharides mustn't distract from produce naturally containing ample fibers. Whole vegetables additionally provide cooperating accessory micronutrients, enzymes and phytochemicals that facilitate symbiosis.

Though yet to become medical standards, clinical indications suggest fermented foods and prebiotic plants do synergize certain antibiotics, mitigate antibiotic-associated diarrhea and enhance cancer immunotherapy outcomes - complementary microbiome-based strategies that avoid devastating dysbiosis side effects of pharmacological options alone.

Potential Probiotic Adjuncts

As introduced earlier, selectively supplementing strains missing within individual microbiomes yet support holistic physiology holds appeal. Alongside prebiotics, live-culture foods may act as vehicles for spore-stable targeted microbes to pass.

Various pathogens coopt wireless communication channels between damaged epithelium and immune cells. This hampers tissue repair signaling. Secreting bioactive metabolites, certain probiotic species may override these blocked frequencies.

For instance, Lactobacillus reuteri, a ubiquitously beneficial species, defaults to shut-down mode without dietary tryptophan yet contributing little to dysbiosis. Animal studies find it restores mucosal regeneration signaling obstructed by Salmonella infections - preventing characteristic diarrhea and translocation-induced sepsis.

Likewise select immunomodulatory soil organisms persist alive through stomach passage when consumed as pills. Mycobacterium vaccae triggers serotonin release through cytokine interaction during stressful contexts- thereby preventing stress-induced intestinal permeability and associated systemic inflammation that depress lymphocytes.

Rather than over-emphasizing isolated probiotic cure-alls, incorporating minimally processed phytonutrient-rich foods containing cooperative microbial diversity alongside any supplemental medicinal flora or fauna holds synergy - the long-standing traditional approach for harmonizing immunity:leveraged ecology, not rigid chemistry alone.

Overall by populating our intestinal ecosystem with beneficial familiar organisms while providing nourishment they and we mutually require for optimal functioning, fermented foods, live cultures and a spectrum of whole plant fibers flexibly sustain favorable biochemical dialogues between microbiome metabolism and human physiology's highest order. Immunity rests upon this evolved, cooperative, multi-kingdom balance flowing through guts and soils alike.

Chapter 7: Healthy Fats, Nuts and Seeds

With carbohydrates and proteins receiving deserved attention for fueling bodily cells, fats strangely endure neglect regarding immune function despite equally vital structural and signaling roles for nearly all physiological processes.

From fueling movement of sentinel immune cells between lymph nodes to constructing eicosanoid inflammatory messengers that coordinate microbial battles, the types of lipids incorporated into cell membranes profoundly influences systemic immune competence - especially response kinetics against recurrent threats.

Nourishing innate defenses through nutritional fat sources high in anti-inflammatory omega-3s, antimicrobial medium-chain triglycerides, bioactive plant sterols and adequately balanced omega-6 arachidonic acid collectively provides raw materials for keeping elaborate lipid-dependent immune components running optimally.

Immunomodulatory Omega-3 Fatty Acids

The discovery that Greenland Inuit populations acquire remarkable cardiovascular protection from omega-3-rich marine oils revealed lipids impart far more than just calories. Beyond bolstering neuronal membranes, omega-3s like EPA/DHA integrate into immune cell phospholipids granting enhanced motility, cytokine flexibility and residential longevity that reduce systemic inflammation driving most modern disease.

Through competitive inhibition, omega-3 incorporation blocks arachidonic acid conversion into pro-inflammatory eicosanoids like tumor-promoting PGE2, platelet-aggregating TXA2 and leukotriene B4 which otherwise perpetuate inflammatory pathogenesis. Resolving signals like lipoxins and protectins generated from DHA also dominate.

These modulating effects meaningfully impact overt inflammatory disorders like asthma and conditions driven by unrestrained inflammation like heart disease, insulin resistance and neurodegeneration- all sharing links to depressed omega-3 levels. Anti-inflammatory benefits likely extend to anxiety, depression and obsessive rumination partially fueled by systemic cytokine imbalance- the true underlying "inflamed mood."

Regularly supplementing bioavailable forms like algal EPA/DHA, krill oil phospholipids or fish oil importantly augments dietary omega-3 intake for individuals subsisting on standard Western diets chronically overfed on omega-6 seed oils. Varied whole food sources further provide bountiful antioxidants and astaxanthin that prevent lipid oxidation.

Antibacterial MCTs from Coconut Oil

The dense medium-chain triglycerides (MCTs) like lauric acid abundantly concentrated within traditional coconut oils and palm kernel emulsions exhibit potent antibacterial, antifungal and antiviral actions against lipid-enveloped microbes by infiltrating membranes.

By displacing rigid cholesterol, introducing fluidity and altering signaling proteins, MCT insertion effectively dissolves viral envelopes and bacterial outer lipid membranes- destroying infectious capacity and unquote viability. This helps prevent infections but likewise clears reservoirs of concealing stealth microbes misidentified as self-tissue by immune cells.

Specific medium-chain fatty acids vigorously challenge dental pathogens like Streptococcus mutans, respiratory colonizers like Haemophilus influenza and numerous intestinal opportunists while also exhibiting anti-parasitic effects against Giardia - promoting gastrointestinal regularity. Whether applied cutaneously, diffuse into sinus passageways, ingested orally or dispersed into room air, MCTs bolster mucus membrane defenses particularly for those prone to hard to eradicate microbial residence.

Coconut derivatives like monolaurin require little processing for cellular absorption compared to elongating long-chain acids, granting more direct antimicrobial benefits. Their versatile everyday applications provide continual reinforcement against persistent lipid-shelled threats that exploit periodic localized epithelial vulnerabilities to drive chronic inflammatory pathogenesis through periodic shedding and systemic dispersal.

Bioactive Vitamin E Complex Tocopherols

Beyond omega fatty acids, vitamin E umbrella tocopherols and tocotrienols concentrate within certain nuts, seeds and leafy plants to prevent lipid oxidation - protecting delicate fats resident within cell membranes and circulating lipoproteins against structural damage by reactive oxygen species that undermine tissue-level function.

However leading immunologists now regard dismissing vitamin E solely as an antioxidant as grossly simplistic given far more profound influences modulating inflammation, apoptosis, platelet aggregation, immune cell differentiation, detoxification capacity, mitochondrial efficiency and lipid storage.

For example, gamma-tocopherol ramps up protective phase II xenobiotic enzymes for enhanced chemical defense and minimizes neutrophil recruitment to injured tissues by attenuating monocyte pro-inflammatory signaling while delta-tocotrienol potently inhibits lipid-sensitive Cox2, 5-Lox and 12-Lox inflammatory enzymes independant of radical scavenging antioxidant capacity.

These multifaceted bioactivities synergize the benefits of ample omega-3 intake, reinforcing balanced inflammatory signaling with antioxidant protection that collectively upholds metabolic and immune integrity- especially among the elderly with accumulating oxidative damage.

Specialized Pro-Resolving Lipid Mediators

Finally unlocking enduring mysteries of self-limited acute inflammation despite perpetual lipid release, pioneering research groups recently characterized a new genre of essential fatty derivatives coined specialized pro-resolving mediators (SPMs) that actively signal inflammatory conclusion.

Powerful nutrients found concentrated in cold water fatty fish and some algae, newly identified docosahexaenoic acid (DHA) metabolites like resolvins, maresins, protectins and lipoxins convey specific molecular instructions for initiating programmed leukocyte death, phagocytic clearance and tissue regeneration once threat neutralization concludes - essentially telling inflammation "you've done your job, now it's time to heal."

By actively resolving inflammation, DHA bioactives prevent unrestrained inflammation underlying countless idiopathic immune conditions. In the context of copious omega-6 and inadequate omega-3 intake driving Western epidemics, supplemental EPA/DHA sources supplying inflammation-resolving SPMs provide a molecular bridge over troubled waters created by physiological imbalance.

Much mystery still swirls around which supplementary nutrients optimally sustain conversion of alpha linoleic acid from nuts and seeds into usable long-chain EPA/DHA that generate these pivotal signaling metabolites - yet eating more anti-inflammatory phytochemicals, fermented foods and bioavailable marine lipids appear beneficial while avoiding omega-6 overconsumption remains imperative.

Through complex dances between nutrient precursors, enzymatic metabolism and lipid-derived signaling molecules interacting with cell receptors, what we eat and digest unavoidably shapes total body homeostasis. Key fatty acids and their derivative compounds provide critical missing links between dietary patterns and modifiable inflammatory processes underlying prevention or progression of most disease states.

Chapter 8: Whole Grains

Beyond just carbohydrate energy sources, intact grains like rice, buckwheat, oats, rye, amaranth and corn furnish diverse bioactive metabolites and fiber types with beneficial immunological activity.

From upregulating intestinal tight junction proteins securing delicate endothelial barriers against allergen and pathogen translocation into circulation to providing sustained fuel for immune cells undergoing rigorous proliferation, minimally refined grains support a multitude of defensive processes in a manner refined flour and sweeteners cannot.

Unfortunately with abundant convenient availability of high glycemic refined grains that lack cooperative accessory nutrients and fiber, intake of balanced slow-burning whole grains continues declining across industrialized nations - corresponding surging gluten sensitivity and poorly manageable weight.

Thankfully incrementally replacing even modest amounts of sugars, white flour products and convenience snacks with more fiber-rich intact whole grains bolsters numerous interdependent physiological processes that collectively enhance disease resilience.

Slow Burn Energy Sustains Immune Cell Proliferation

Upon recognizing foreign antigens, lymphocytes promptly activate and undergo intense metabolic activity to rapidly clone specific cell lines equipped for custom counter offense. This burst of new cells requires substantial energy to fuel growth and specialized production of antibodies, chemical messengers and cytotoxic proteins.

High glycemic carbohydrates cause rapid blood sugar spikes that trigger equally rapid crashes which fail to provide sustained energy for racing lymphocytes - compared to fibrous whole grains that slowly drip-feed gentler supply of encased glucose molecules over hours without dramatic peaks and dips.

Smooth steady glucose delivery optimizes conditions for emerging lymphocytes to mature into fully armed battalions before exhausting initial fuel reserves. Without wavering energy, adequate nutrients and growth receptors, fledgling immune cells perish before completing rigorous bootcamp transformation. Sustained slow-burn carb sources help ensure sufficient gasoline reaches frontline medic troops summoned at a moment's notice no matter the hour.

Bioactive Metabolites Improve Detoxification

Beyond pure macronutrition, whole grains like quinoa contain unique bioactive saponins that exhibit direct antibacterial properties by permeating outer cell membranes at the site of infectious threat. Additional grain compounds enhance endogenous detoxification capacity to clear accrued toxic metabolites that would otherwise provoke inflammation and derail immune cell duties.

Avenanthramides exclusive to oats demonstrate anti-inflammatory, anti-itch and antioxidant activity by suppressing histamine release from agitated mast cells characteristic of eczema and urticaria. Rye and wheat bran contain phenolic amides that upregulate glutathione production to combat free radicals while eliciting cancer cell death.

Boosting liver enzymes that tag toxins for disposal supports immunosurveillance duties minimizing collateral damage from chemical exposures that undermine immune cell regeneration and detox processes necessary for managing increasing man-made environmental challenges ubiquitous to modern living.

Choosing whole grains over refined imposters thereby furnishes physiological systems multiple accessory allies against numerous antagonists while providing pure fuel for the enduring metabolic intensity of adaptive cell expansion.

Prebiotic Fibers Selectively Feed Protective Bugs

Grain components also supply a bounty of fibers and resistant starches that pass undigested through small intestines into the colon where hungry resident commensals like Bifidobacterium selectively prosper and reward us in return with invaluable immune programming signals.

Certain whole grain phenolic metabolites even exhibit selective antimicrobial actions against dangerous fungi like Candida albicans found provoking intestinal permeability and systemic inflammation among the inappropriate antibiotic exposure, chronic stress and sugar consumption endemic to modern societies.

Through both substrate support for binding good guys and direct inhibition of hazardous opportunists by grain protective compounds, frequent consumption of minimally processed intact whole grains translates into greater microbiome richness and reinforced mucosal integrity vital for kept for managing heightened modern antigenic load - sustaining resilience.

Anti-Inflammatory Short-Chain Fatty Acid Metabolites

As introduced earlier, beneficial saccharolytic bacteria like Roseburia, Eubacterium and Faecalibacterium species possess specialized enzymes to unlock and feast upon certain resistant starches and prebiotic fibers that human metabolism cannot directly access.

In exchange for these gifts of difficult yet abundantly available dietary plant substrates, symbionts share short-chain fatty acid metabolites like beneficial butyrate with intestinal cells and immune regulatory cells that calibrate homeostasis.

Constant crosstalk through receptors situated along intestinal lining allows lymph and blood cell components continually sample these bacterial fermentation byproducts for gauging current environmental immunological status. The consequently modified signaling patterns go on to set systemic tone balancing tolerance against attack.

This means the variable microbiome population flux and their preferential metabolic output directly instructs host immune homeostasis. Hence "you are what your microbes eat" - supported directly by eating more anti-inflammatory prebiotic whole grains that ultimately feeds us.

Chapter 9: Legumes and Lean Proteins

While overtly supporting immune vigor may not seem an obvious application for beans, lentils and lean animal proteins, these savory dietary staples provide vital amino acids for renewing the elaborate protein structures that comprise antibodies, cytokines, receptors, enzymes and structural scaffolding vital for lymphocytes to effectively neutralize threats.

Worse still, without adequate lean protein continually replenishing aged and damaged tissues, the cumulative effects of old injuries and microbial fragments linger generating antigenic debris for which tolerance fails prompting attacks against self. Thus sufficient daily protein prevents autoimmunity.

However, not all dietary protein sources furnish equal immunological benefit. Certain legumes and unprocessed animal flesh enhance resilience while others provoke inflammation that sabotages defense efforts. Discerning optimal choices remains imperative. Let's survey immune impacts of various proteins.

Amino Acids - Bioactive Building Blocks

During active threats, rapidly proliferating B and T cell lymphocytes require abundant amino acids to mass produce specialized antibodies and cell killing proteins. Cysteine constitutes a rate limiting substrate for endogenous antioxidant glutathione synthesis while glutamine fuels gut barrier integrity to restrict allergen flux.

Both bone broth soups and marinated baked tempeh provide all essential amino acids for combating infection including sulfur amino acids that counter pain signaling and phase II liver detox enzymes which clear drug metabolites that would otherwise provoke organ stress and systemic inflammation that distracts active immune processes.

Phase appropriate protein intake enables fabrication of critical components that identifies threats for attentive lymphocytes while preventing loss of self-tolerance and resultant autoimmunity from accumulating debris of defective constituents.

Lean Clean Proteins Aid Detoxification

Beyond basic nutrition, certain amino configurations also signal biological pathways to assist detoxification of chemical exposures nearly ubiquitous to modern life that disrupt DNA repair processes and healing.

Glutathione synthesis depends on cysteine availability while glycine rich collagen upregulates phase II hepatic enzymes that attach electron donating groups on stored environmental toxins and pharmaceutical metabolites to ease elimination and prevent bioaccumulative inflammatory damage.

Eating wild caught anchovies, organ meats, whey protein and vegetables like okra provides favorable building blocks that sustains the elaborate architecture empire underlying our intrinsic healing processes.

Concentrated chemical toxins store within animal fat cells and visceral adipose. Lean clean flesh from wild caught fish, pasture raised fowl and grassfed ruminants avoid concentrated environmental pollutants and inflammatory saturated fats prevalent in conventional meat that undermine immune efforts.

Anti-Inflammatory Plant Proteins

Beyond animal flesh, certain legumes and grains offer beneficial plant proteins without pro-inflammatory risks of disruptive persistent chemicals accrued across lengthy food chains subject to bioaccumulation.

Sprouted brown rice protein contains balancing serotonin precursors to offset stress-induced immune changes while chickpeas offer bioavailable amino acids absent the common sensitivities of allergenic gluten and dairy - providing steady nourishment during illness recovery periods of heightened protein demand that challenges digestion.

Fermented soybean-derived tempeh offers complete proteins including genistein that help counter inflammation underlying chronic infection mechanisms that exploit periodic intestinal vulnerability. Lentils furnish zinc and iron to facilitate hundreds of metalloenzyme immune processes.

Consuming abundant plant proteins avoids downstream consequences of commercial meat production like shifted intestinal microbiota and reduced colonic mucus thickness that predictably trigger permeability and food sensitivity. Thus plant and clean animal proteins synergize resilience.

Immunosupportive Micronutrient Minerals

Trace dietary minerals like zinc, selenium and magnesium activate elaborate enzymatic cascades that structure lymph tissue development and effective threat response signaling self destruct programs in cancerous cells.

Zinc concentrates within thymic tissue maturing T helper cells while boosting dendritic cell antigen presentation, natural killer cell cytotoxicity and restraining mast cell histamine release.

Selenium antioxidants prevent lipid peroxidation in cell membranes protecting structural integrity while contributing vital cofactors for glutathione enzymes used in quenching free radicals.

Magnesium salts draw fluids for immune cells to migrate toward pathogens across endothelial barriers into injured tissues which then uptake the mineral to begin proliferative repair phases.

These three critical minerals concentrate within grains, legumes, nuts and unpolluted seafood - foods that both provide building blocks for restoring health while enhancing the elaborate cleanup processes required to resolve inflammatory conditions toward homeostasis.

Chapter 10: Foods High in Vitamins and Minerals

As introduced in earlier sections, certain vitamins and minerals serve as vital enzymatic cofactors underlying intricate molecular machinery powering immune cell duties. Though only required in trace quantities, deficiencies or imbalance among such key micronutrients predictably undermine various defense processes.

Conversely, consuming vitamin and mineral rich foods trains physiology towards heightened disease resistance by ensuring lymphocyte proliferation, microbial targeting and critical cleanup roles proceed unencumbered by accidental deprived substrate scarcity that might delay crucial response timelines.

Many enzyme-driven processes like quenching liver detox byproducts require specific rare helpers found concentrated in select animal and plant based foods evolved to furnish physiological systems elements needed for combating dynamic environmental threats aimed at host assimilation and exploitation. Let's survey key immunity vitamins and minerals along with their dietary sources.

Vitamin C

Fruits and vegetables naturally concentrate various critical immune cofactors. For example citrus, peppers, crucifers and leafy greens provide abundant antioxidant vitamin C shown clinically to shorten duration of cold symptoms by supporting interferon-driven antiviral mechanisms as well as neutrophil pathogen clearance while preserving endogenous glutathione stores.

Primates uniquely lost the enzyme to internally synthesize potent vitamin C unlike nearly all other mammals, likely explaining humanity's peculiar susceptibilities to scurvy and infection. Yet nature graciously provides abundant external sources like oranges, mangos, papaya, kiwi, red bell peppers, broccoli, parsley and herbal rose hips.

Adequate Vitamin C also enables synthesis of collagen extracellular matrix proteins necessary for tissue repair after immune battles degrade damaged cells into debris requiring removal for full resolution back into homeostasis.

Vitamin D

Though technically a prohormonal steroid, activated vitamin D fits criteria for an immunomodulatory micronutrient obtained through sunlight exposure yet also concentrated in certain animal foods naturally high in fat soluble nutrients like oily fish, fish roe, eggs and beef liver.

Vitamin D crucially upholds tight junctions sealing off intestinal and lung epithelial layers to infectious threats which attempt access into circulation to spread systemically. This barrier protection combined with enhancing antimicrobial peptide secretion explains much of the clinical efficacy of Vitamin D against respiratory infections and supplemented protection against autoimmunity.

However safe sun exposure remains ideal for those with sufficient melanin to avoid burning while responsibly sourced eggs, wild caught salmon and cheese offer some dietary vitamin D that further supports immune functioning dependent on this multipurpose ingredient so uniquely synthesized through direct solar-energized transformation of skin oils.

Vitamin A

Similarly found abundantly in colorful antioxidant-rich plants, vitamin A as colorful carotenoids convert into active retinal needed for night vision yet also supports mucosal barriers lining respiratory and digestive passages- preventing infectious penetration.

These vivid fat soluble phytochemicals concentrate within liver, egg yolks and dairy cream as retinol more readily used by cells to reinforce membrane junctions sealing out threats. Active vitamin A also expedites apoptosis and promotes regulatory T-cell differentiation- preventing excessive delayed reactions that enable chronic pathology.

Vitamin A further activates macrophages while acutely suppressing neutrophil recruitment reducing collateral damage into resolution phases of controlled inflammation- effectively handing off healing responsibilities to proliferative reconstruction cells after eliminating instigating irritants. Carrot, sweet potato, spinach and cod liver oil furnish dietary vitamin A.

Zinc

As introduced earlier, bioavailable trace minerals like zinc activate hundreds of enzymatic processes vital for nucleic acid metabolism and intracellular communication underlying lymphocyte actions against pathogens. High zinc foods like oysters, beef, pumpkin seeds, shitake mushrooms and sea vegetables provide up to 30% daily value per serving.

Beyond basic nutrition, certain amino configurations also signal biological pathways to assist detoxification of chemical exposures nearly ubiquitous to modern life that disrupt DNA repair processes and healing.

Iron

Meats and spinach offer heme iron most easily absorbed to deliver oxygen while beans, nuts and whole grains provide plant-based iron that buffers absorption rates to prevent uncontrolled oxidative stress from too much too quick accumulation of volatile ferrous ions. Both forms bind oxygen essential for metabolically active infection-fighting white blood cells.

Iron further enables creation of free radical intermediates unleashed from innate immune cells against invading threats which are further quenched by antioxidant rich foods preventing excessive inflammation to surrounding tissues. Together with zinc and vitamin A, iron allows for coordinated anti-pathogen offensive measures.

Selenium

Concentrated in a few selenium-accumulator plants like mushrooms and brazil nuts, this essential dietary trace mineral forms a key constituent of endogenous antioxidant enzymes glutathione peroxidase and thioredoxin reductase-both critically limiting inflammatory lipid peroxidation and DNA mutations from free radical pathology while recycling oxidized vitamin C back into active form.

Selenium supplementation shows profound immune stimulation, enhancing neutrophil superoxide bursts used against pathogens. Brace nuts alone providing 700% RDA per ounce. Intelligent supplementation therefore bolsters antioxidant capacity vital to resolving inflammatory collateral damage.

On the whole by directly providing vital phytochemicals while concentrating rare but essential micronutrients into bioavailable forms, certain functional foods selectively support myriad molecular processes underlying optimal immune surveillance, signaling and clearance duties- allowing cells to effectively quench microbial and malignant threats.

Adequate vitamin and mineral sources furnish indigenous physiology abundant raw materials needed for fabricating vast diversity of proteins, enzymes, messengers and receptors essential for maintained smooth function across interdependent systems that sustain our health and survival.

Part III: The Immune-Boosting Eating Plan

Having explored the intricate workings of the immune system, we now shift our focus to practical application. In this section, we present an integrated dietary framework designed to fortify the immune system, translating scientific insights into everyday food choices that enhance resilience.

Consider this evidence-based meal guidance as your field manual, strategically incorporating nutritious foods to strengthen your health defense arsenal. The emphasis is on traditional whole foods from diverse cultures, supplemented intelligently when modern circumstances hinder the consumption of fermented foods, phytochemical-rich plants, and clean proteins. This approach aims to provide a varied spectrum of nutrients that feed intricate biochemical pathways crucial for holistic health.

The dietary recommendations are adaptable to personal preferences and tolerances while considering the general needs of a healthy population. Individuals dealing with complex conditions may require additional considerations, but the foundational principles remain universally applicable for preventing the impact of inflammatory lifestyle factors and building resistance against chronic diseases.

Cultivating resilience goes beyond mere protection, focusing on bouncing back quickly in case pathogens breach defenses. The guidelines provided here aim to offer daily nutrition that fuels critical healing mechanisms, supporting both avoidance and rapid recovery during sickness.

Regular exposure to fermented foods provides continuous immune training, helping recognize harmless compounds for tolerance development. A diverse array of plant foods furnishes phytochemicals and prebiotics that feed commensal species, which, in turn, reciprocate with critical metabolites. Carefully chosen animal and seafood proteins provide balanced nourishment, contributing to the fabrication of an elaborate architecture that protects health.

The goal is to unlock your inner healing potential through an evolutionarily approved eating strategy, activating formidable defenses. It's time to feed your immune system and embrace a holistic approach to health.

Chapter 11: Designing Your Immune-Supportive Diet

While some marketing claims irresponsibly promise miracle cures from isolated compounds, genuine immune nourishment relies on evidence-based holistic strategies that feed interdependent defensive systems through synergistic combinations of whole traditional foods selected by ancestral logic.

There exist no singular silver bullet herbs, nutrients or health products capable of enhancing such profound multidimensional physiology in isolation. Authentic solutions come through cooperating with biology, not dictating against it. To meet layered defense needs from resilient barriers to pathogen clearance and balanced immunological tolerance, nutrition must nourish systems at every interacting level.

The following guidelines integrate past and present science on preventing dysfunction while providing raw materials to enhance innate healing processes when conditions progress beyond initial stages of avoidance. These universal recommendations serve as templates for customization based on individual needs.

Eat The Rainbow Every Day

Abundant deeply pigmented antioxidant-rich whole fruits and vegetables provide a solid nutritional foundation by furnishing vast phytochemical variety supporting cellular repair processes that counter inflammation and free radical damage that distracts immune duties.

Each vivid color group like red berries and purple plums concentrates distinct bioactive compounds with specialized activities. For example orange pumpkin and carrots offer carotenoids to enhance night vision and bolster mucus membrane barriers while indoles in cruciferous broccoli and cabbage assist liver detoxification.

Beyond championing any single "superfood" fruits or vegetables, strive for spectrum diversity across meals to obtain range of polyphenols, carotenoids and antioxidants that concentrate uniquely across plant groups based on evolutionary roles attracting pollinators, defending against pests and healing from foraging damage.

Choose organic whenever possible to avoid concentrated agrochemicals that impair natural detox processes. Fermenting cabbage into antioxidant rich sauerkraut and kimchi or sprouting sunflower greens from whole seeds boosts innate phytochemicals and friendly microbes that confer mucosal protection from seasonal allergies.

Emphasize Anti-Inflammatory Foods

Chronic inflammation sabotages physiological functioning by perpetuating cell danger signaling cascades that disrupt tissue repair processes. Without active resolution, persistent inflammation inevitably causes cumulative breakdown interfering with routine immune duties – allowing opportunistic pathogens to exploit periodic vulnerabilities initiating downward spiral as symptoms compound.

Frequently sampling edibles shown to resolve inflammatory pathways allows innate processes to restore balanced functioning. Anti-inflammatory foods include oily cold water fish, bright citrus fruits, tart cherry juice, turmeric root, green tea, garlic, berries, dark greens, mushrooms, papaya, apple cider vinegar, bone broth soups and bioavailable curcumin supplements.

Each unique food concentrates specialized metabolites that interface with particular inflammatory signals – cumulatively targeting the common underlying nucleus of most chronic hypometabolic diseases. Amplifying a spectrum of signals that conclude unnecessary inflammation saves physiology from squandering irreplaceable resources against false threats, freeing function to flourish.

Nourish The Microbiome

Teeming communities of symbiont bacteria residing along intestinal villi profoundly direct appropriate immune education, threatened response signaling and inflammatory counter-regulation through dynamic molecular crosstalk along epithelial borders. These commensal microbe populations rely entirely on dietary substrates for their specialized metabolic outputs that train systemic immunity.

Cultivating rich "good guy" diversity through intake of divers fiber-rich whole food carbohydrates– especially fermented grains, traditional dairy, raw honey and perennial roots like yams – provides sustained nourishment that yields anti-inflammatory metabolites which beneficially calibrate homeostasis against modern dysbiotic pressures.

Probiotic supplements show context-specific upside in recolonizing specific commensal species with known beneficial secretions that remain depleted in disorders with characteristic microbiome defects. Yet supplements alone prove no substitute for continual dietary nourishment and immune training via minimally heated naturally cultured foods containing rich cooperative microbial diversity – the ultimate plan for sustaining genetic wealth.

Emphasize Foods Over Supplements

Isolated nutrients, herbs or nutraceutical extracts support specific pathways, but often disappoint through nuanced collaborative human chemistry. Whereas cultures subsisting on balanced whole food cuisine through seasonal native plants, fermented grains and sustainable animal proteins remain largely free of degenerative diseases – whereas Americans perish from systemic inflammation despite trillions spent on healthcare and condition-specific supplements.

Obviously no single compound substitutes for foundational lifestyle nutrition choices that nourish interconnected systems simultaneously. Yet targeted supplements judiciously applied can helpfully tune certain phenotypic expressions gone awry when modern environments introduce novel xenobiotics, stressors and foods that mismatch intrinsic needs evolved over millennia.

Responsibly applying protective or regenerative supplements around foundational wholesome balanced ingestion of recognizable traditional foods braces physiology for modernity, whereas supplements alone prove structurally incapable of fulfilling layered nutritional deficit created by postmodern convenience consumption patterns.

Reduce Pro-Inflammatory Edibles

Equally important as increasing anti-inflammatory and immunosupportive foods remains eliminating dietary contributors that suppress immunity or fuel inflammation antagonizing intricate molecular signaling regulating homeostasis and repair processes.

Abundant omega 6 oils, refined grains with isolated sugars, chemicalized factory farm meat, artificial additives and pesticide residue all undermine defensible resilience by distracting critical processes. Less dietary disturbances grants focused resources for enhancing important layered microbial communities and endogenous metabolic pathways that regenerate and uphold holistic wellbeing.

Protective nutrition proves foundational across prevention and therapeutic spectra – whether avoiding dysfunction downstream or correcting pathology already expressing. Eliminating antagonists improves outcomes regardless of particular condition specifics while adding supportive foods becomes highly individualized by unique genotype, lifestyle and environmental exposures that tune phenotypic disease manifestation.

Nutrients Depend On Food Matrix Chemistry

Prefer whole food sources over synthesized vitamins whenever viable for enhanced phytonutrient bioavailability and nutrient carriage. The fibrous cellular structures housing vitamins in nature elegantly buffer absorption kinetics to ideal sustained delivery rates as foods pass through gastric phases - whereas compacted isolated fractions alarm digestive lining signaling rapid wholesale transport, straining homeostatic balance.

Further, the elaborate symphony of accessory micronutrients and phytochemicals cooperating with primary ingredients within whole foods participates extensively in metabolic break down, directing synergistic delivery or variable contingent pathways based on current physiological need signals.

These graceful feedback loops remain silenced in solitary molecules presented against an empty biological stage – lacking nuanced support for transport, signaling, metabolism and excretion after serving necessitous functions within particular cells and tissues. Holistic nourishment proves far more than consuming bulk assumed substrate amounts alone.

Customize Selections To Your Needs

General recommendations provide helpful templates for modifying into personalized plans based on individual genotypes, lifestyle factors and health goals. Customizing food choices to your unique demands enables precision nutrition rather than blanket recommendations that inadequately address layered variables comprising whole circumstance.

For example, those with autoimmunity and alley or digestive disorders likely demand specialized elimination approaches compared to athletes requiring maximum muscle fuels for intense training regimens under high oxidative stress.

Ancestral clues embedded within cultural cuisine provide hints at ideal staples for particular backgrounds that sustainably nourish associated genotypes evolved over generations. Yet deviations still exist even between genetic twins, arguing further customization. Inputs from blood panels assessing clotting factors, cholesterol efflux capability, CRP and nutrient status better inform precision adjustments.

No universal guidelines reliably apply equally to all people given vast biochemical individuality. Fortunately, foundational principles support beneficial modification into customized plans optimized for your unique demands.

Structure Meals Around Macronutrients

Regardless of personalized food selections, structurally categorizing daily intake volumes based on optimal macronutrient distribution ranges enhances consistency meeting estimated biological needs for average healthy populations with moderate activity levels.

Whether satisfying these nourishing ratios through plants or animals remains elective for individuals to test based on genomic heritage, ethical dietary preferences, culture, access and health goals. Yet universally, moderate protein with lower glycemic carbohydrates, high antioxidant wholefood fats and abundant anti-inflammatory fiber benefits most by preventing inflammation and metabolic disturbances that divert immune duties.

General macronutrient ratio guidance for structurally balancing meals follow:

20-30% Daily Calories from Protein (80-120g for 2000 cal)

30-45% Daily Calories from Carbohydrate (150-225g for 2000 cal) with emphasis on vegetables > fruits > whole intact grains > minimal added sugar

25-50% Daily Calories from Fat (55-110g for 2000 cal) with emphasis on omega-3s > monounsaturated > omega-6 vegetable oils

Minimum 30g Fiber from mixed wholefood sources

Testing various personalized ratios within these general guidelines through meal plans structured around macronutrients proves vital for optimizing gene expression potentials tuned through nourishment.

Incorporate Intermittent Fasting

Beyond base nutrition calculations, emerging science confirms gene expression and metabolic processes that control subjective appetite craving, fat burning efficiency, and inflammatory regulation dynamically fluctuate based on eating frequency patterns relative to daily cycles of sleep, sun exposure, movement and stress. This innate biological rhythm steers physiology through nourishing phases of tissue rebuilding, energy storage and cellular cleanup processes across days and seasons.

Intermittent fasting through periodic partial day reduction in meal frequency or caloric intake supports metabolic homeostasis by allowing overnight repair intervals of stimulated autophagy processes to clear damaged proteins and organelles without constant digestion demands diverting vital resources.

This inherent intermittent biohazard remediation period concentrates turnover and renewal operations into targeted bursts through day/night cycling - upholding cellular order against entropy dynamics. Regular fasting intervals by simply limiting nighttime eating and snacks to allow deeper overnight cleansing fasts supports innate metabolic cycles structurally rooted in circadian biology since antiquity.

Structure Nutrition Around Lifestyle Demands

Finally, tailoring nutritional plans to complement periodic demands from unique lifestyle factors like competitive athletics, intensities of physical training, cognitive performance needs and stressful work projects better equips defined physiology for spurts of increased requirements that flux based on day to day goals and challenges through phases of growth and renewal.

For example, strength building requires additional protein before and after resistance exercise to supply available substrate fractions for new muscle protein synthesis during subsequent nightly repair processes - whereas cognitive tasks depend more on consistent glucose from lower glycemic carbohydrate metabolism and enhanced blood flow from dietary nitrates that concentrate in beets and leafy greens.

Like a well-conducted orchestra, each section of nutritional selection should synchronize appropriately to meet peaking needs during key moments of business across interconnected metabolic systems that collectively support holistic aims underlying lifestyle demands.

This integrated timing approach to eating for defined purposes based on informed understanding of interconnected biological processes supports enhanced performance while also identifying overconsumption that fuels dysfunction. Quality nutrition aligns to serve greater collective purposes rather than chasing momentary cravings alone independent of long-view intent.

Chapter 12: Recipes to Feed Your Defenses

Applying evidence-based meal guidance from the previous nutrition-focused chapters, this section features 28 diverse globally inspired recipes centered around traditional whole foods selected for their multifaceted support of total body systems that collectively underlie resilient immune defenses.

Beyond general healthy eating, these dishes emphasize anti-inflammatory edibles, phytochemical richness, microbe nourishing ferments, metabolic balancing macronutrient ratios and synergistic food combinations designed specifically to nourish intricate processes regulating innate disease resistance and sustained wellbeing.

While not medical prescriptions, incorporates science-backed principles through palate-pleasing preparations you can integrate into regular rotation based on seasonal availability, cost factors and personal preferences. Feel free to creatively modify based on unique needs.

This home kitchen friendly selection intends to inspire lasting behavioral change through enjoyable culinary exploration that cooperates with, rather than dictates against, evolved human biochemistry for punctuated nourishment around lifestyle demands. Now let's feed formidable defenses through flaming feast!

Rainbow Salad with Tamari Ginger Dressing

- 1/2 head red cabbage, shredded

- 2 carrots, cut into thin strips

- 1 beet, peeled and grated

- 1 mango, peeled, pitted and diced

- 1 avocado, peeled, pitted and diced

- 1 cup cooked chickpeas

- 1/4 cup tahini

- 3 Tbsp rice vinegar

- 1 inch ginger, minced

- 2 Tbsp tamari

- 1 tsp toasted sesame oil

- 1 lime, juiced

- 1/4 tsp garlic powder

- Salt and pepper to taste

- Whisk tahini, tamari, vinegar, oil, ginger, lime juice and garlic powder until smooth consistency sauce forms. Thin with water to reach desired drizzle consistency.

- Mix cabbage, carrots, beet, mango, avocado and chickpeas gently in large bowl.

- Drizzle desired amount of dressing over salad just before eating and enjoy!

Tropical Fruit Smoothie

- 1 banana, frozen

- 1 cup pineapple, frozen

- 1 cup coconut water

- 1 cup spinach

- 1 Tbsp flaxseed meal

- 1 tsp baobab powder

- 1 tsp maca powder

- 1 tsp turmeric powder

- 1/2 inch ginger, minced

- 1/2 lemon, juiced

- Ice cubes to blend

- Add all ingredients into high powered blender.

- Blend until smooth consistency reached.

- Enjoy this refreshing vibrant elixir!

Overnight Steel Cut Oats

- 1/2 cup steel cut oats

- 1 1/2 cups nut milk

- 1/4 cup yogurt

- 1 Tbsp chia seeds

- 1 tsp cinnamon

- 1 tsp vanilla

- 1 pinch salt

- Fresh fruit to top

- Mix all ingredients besides fruit into a container.

- Refrigerate overnight until thickened to preferred texture.

- Top with your choice of fruit before enjoying. Consider berries, bananas, mango or persimmon.

Loaded Baked Sweet Potato

- 2 medium sweet potatoes

- 1 15-ounce can black beans, rinsed and drained

- 1 avocado, diced

- 1/4 cup salsa

- 2 Tbsp pumpkin seeds

- 1 lime, juiced

- 1/4 cup cilantro, chopped

- Preheat oven to 425°F. Pierce potatoes with fork, place directly on oven rack and bake 45-60 minutes until fork slides easily through flesh.

- Slice potatoes down the center. Fluff insides with fork and top with beans, avocado, salsa, seeds, cilantro and lime juice.

Curried Lentil Soup

- 1 cup dried green or brown lentils

- 1 onion, diced

- 3 carrots, sliced

- 3 celery stalks, chopped

- 1 inch ginger, minced

- 3 garlic cloves, minced

- 1 Tbsp curry powder

- 6 cups vegetable broth

- 14 oz can coconut milk

- 2 cups spinach

- lime wedges, for serving

- cilantro, for garnish

- Rinse lentils. In large pot over medium heat, sauté onion, carrots, celery, ginger and garlic for 5 minutes until softened.

- Stir in curry powder followed by broth and lentils. Simmer uncovered for 25 minutes, until lentils soften.

- Remove 2 cups broth and purée with coconut milk. Return to pot and stir together.

- Add spinach and cook additional 5 minutes until leaves wilt.

- Serve into bowls garnished with cilantro and lime wedges.

Carrot Bacon

- 12 large carrots, peeled

- 6 Tbsp tamari

- 1 Tbsp maple syrup

- 1 tsp smoked paprika

- 1 tsp garlic powder

- 1/2 tsp onion powder

- 1/2 tsp salt

- Preheat oven 400°F. Line large baking sheet with parchment.

- Slice carrots lengthwise into 1/4 inch planks. Place in single layer on sheet.

- Whisk tamari, syrup and spices. Brush mixture evenly coating carrots.

- Bake 20 minutes, flip and brush again, bake 20 additional minutes until browned and slightly crisped but still tender inside.

Green Breakfast Tacos

- 8 corn tortillas

- 1 15-ounce can black beans, drained and rinsed

- 2 cups spinach

- 1 avocado, sliced

- 1 mango, diced

- 2 green onions, diced

- 1/2 cup salsa verde

- Hot sauce, to taste

- Warm tortillas in dry pan over medium heat.

- In bowl, mix black beans, spinach, avocado, mango and green onions.

- Assembly tacos by evenly dividing bean mixture between tortillas.

- Top with salsa verde and hot sauce. Fold and enjoy!

Pineapple Kimchi Fried Rice

- 3 cups cooked brown rice

- 2 carrots, diced

- 1 onion, diced

- 1 red bell pepper, diced

- 3 eggs, scrambled

- 1 cup kimchi

- 2 green onions, sliced

- 1 cup pineapple, diced

- 1 Tbsp sesame oil

- 2 Tbsp tamari

- Sesame seeds to garnish

- Heat oil in large skillet or wok over medium high heat.

- Add carrots, onion and red pepper. Sauté for 2 minutes.

- Add rice and kimchi. Continue sautéing 3 more minutes.

- Push rice mixture to sides. Add eggs and scramble until just cooked, then combine with rice.

- Add green onions, pineapple and tamari. Sauté additional 2 minutes until fully incorporated.

- Serve garnished with sesame seeds. Enjoy!

Mediterranean Baked Salmon

- 4 salmon fillets

- 1 lemon, sliced

- 1/2 cup kalamata olives, pitted and halved

- 1 pint cherry tomatoes, halved

- 4 cloves garlic, minced

- 2 Tbsp fresh oregano, chopped

- Optional fresh dill

- Olive oil

- Salt and pepper

- Preheat oven to 400°F. Line baking dish with parchment paper.

- Place salmon skin-side down and top with sliced lemons, olives, tomatoes, garlic, oregano and optional dill.

- Drizzle olive oil generously over top and season with salt and pepper.

- Bake 12-15 minutes until salmon flakes easily with fork.

- Serve lemon slices on the side and enjoy this omega-3 rich dish!

Purple Cauliflower Tabouli Salad

- 2 cups quinoa, cooked

- 1 large head purple cauliflower, finely chopped

- 1 pint grape tomatoes, halved

- 1 English cucumber, diced

- 1 cup Italian parsley, chopped

- 1/2 cup fresh mint leaves, chopped

- 1/4 cup olive oil

- 3 Tbsp lemon juice

- 1 lemon, zested

- 2 garlic cloves, minced

- 1 tsp sea salt

- Romaine lettuce cups

- In large bowl, mix together quinoa, cauliflower, tomatoes, cucumber, parsley and mint leaves.

- In small bowl, whisk together olive oil, lemon juice, lemon zest, garlic and salt.

- Add dressing to salad and stir thoroughly to coat.

- Serve chilled or room temperature into romaine lettuce cups or over spinach bed.

Cranberry Orange Immune Elixir

- 4 cups water

- 1 cup fresh cranberries

- 1 orange, peeled and sliced

- 1 apple, cored and sliced

- 1/4 cup cranberries, honey

- 1/4 tsp powdered ginger

- 1/4 tsp powdered cinnamon

- Pinch cayenne pepper

- Add water, cranberries, orange, apple, honey and spices to medium pot.

- Bring to a boil, then reduce heat and simmer 20 minutes.

- Remove from heat and allow to slightly cool 15 minutes.

- Pour through fine mesh strainer into pitcher, using spoon to crush fruit against strainer for maximum juice extraction.

- Discard pulp. Chill elixir before serving. Sip this vibrant potion through the day!

Curry Butternut Squash Soup

- 1 large butternut squash, about 4 cups chopped flesh

- 1 onion, chopped

- 2 carrots, chopped

- 1 Granny Smith apple, peeled and chopped

- 1 inch fresh ginger, minced

- 2 Tbsp olive oil

- 2 Tbsp Thai red curry paste

- 6 cups vegetable broth

- 14 fl. oz. full-fat coconut milk

- Juice of 1 lime

- 1/4 cup fresh cilantro, chopped

- Heat oil over medium heat in large stockpot. Add onion, carrots, apple and ginger. Sauté for 5 minutes until softened.

- Add squash and continue cooking additional 5 minutes, stirring occasionally.

- Add curry paste and stir constantly 1 minute to bloom spices.

- Pour in broth, submerging vegetables. Raise heat and bring to boil.

- Reduce heat, cover and simmer 25 minutes until squash easily mashes with fork or spoon against pot edge.

- Remove from heat. Purée half the soup at a time in blender, returning to pot.

- Stir in coconut milk and lime juice. Adjust consistency if needed with additional broth.

- Serve bowls garnished with fresh cilantro.

Green Shakshuka

- 1 yellow onion, chopped

- 1 jalapeño, seeded and chopped

- 3 garlic cloves, minced

- 1 cup spinach

- 1 cup kale leaves, chopped

- 1 cup frozen peas

- 6 eggs

- 28 oz can diced tomatoes

- 1 lime, juiced

- 1/2 cup feta cheese, crumbled

- Chopped cilantro

- Hot sauce

- Heat deep skillet over medium. Sauté onion, jalapeño and garlic 3 minutes.

- Add spinach, kale and peas. Continue cooking until wilted.

- With spoon, make 6 wells nestled within vegetables. Crack 1 egg into each well.

- Pour tomatoes evenly over top with lime juice and season with salt and pepper. Cover and cook 8 minutes for runny yolks or longer for firmer eggs.

- Remove lid, sprinkle with feta and cilantro. Serve with hot sauce.

Almond Truffles

- 1 cup raw almonds

- 3/4 cup pitted Medjool dates

- 2 Tbsp almond butter

- 1 Tbsp coconut oil, melted

- 1/2 tsp vanilla extract

- 1/4 cup cacao powder

- 1/4 cup shredded unsweetened coconut

- Process almonds in food processor into fine meal with some larger chunks remaining. Transfer almond flour to mixing bowl.

- Add dates, almond butter, coconut oil and vanilla to food processor. Process until smooth consistency dough forms, about 2 minutes.

- Mix cacao powder into almond meal. Roll tablespoon sized date dough balls through meal until evenly coated all around.

- Spread coconut flakes on small plate. Roll each ball through flakes to adhere final coating layer.

- Store finished truffles in airtight container for grab and go sweet tooth satisfaction!

Golden Milk

- 2 cups almond milk

- 1 Tbsp ghee or coconut oil

- 2 Tbsp honey or maple syrup

- 1 Tbsp turmeric powder

- 1 tsp cinnamon

- 1/2 tsp ginger powder

- 1/4 tsp cardamom

- Pinch black pepper

- Pinch cayenne pepper

- Whisk all ingredients except milk in small saucepan over medium heat until warmed through and spices infuse oils. About 2 minutes

- Add milk slowly while whisking briskly to fully incorporate spices, bringing just to a gentle simmer.

- Transfer spiced milk to blender, cover with lid slightly ajar. Blend 30 seconds until frothy.

- Pour into mugs and sip this anti-inflammatory elixir!

Purple Sweet Potato Gnocchi

- 2 large purple sweet potatoes, baked

- 1 cup almond flour

- 2 eggs

- 1 tsp garlic powder

- 1/2 tsp nutmeg

- 1 Tbsp olive oil

- 2 cups marinara sauce

- Scoop cooled sweet potato flesh into mixing bowl. Mash until smooth, then add almond flour, eggs and spices. Fold gently just until incorporated dough ball forms.

- On well floured surface, divide dough into 4 equal pieces. Roll each piece into long 1/2 inch diameter logs.

- Use bench scraper or knife to cut logs crosswise into 1/2 inch pieces. Roll cut pieces gently down tines of a fork, imprinting lines on both sides while slightly flattening.

- Bring large pot of salted water to boil. Add gnocchi pieces and simmer only until all floating pieces rise back up to surface. Do not overcook!

- Drain immediately into serving bowls. Toss gnocchi gently with olive oil to prevent sticking. Top with warm marinara sauce.

Pho Bone Broth

- 3 pounds beef marrow bones

- 1 onion, halved

- 1 inch ginger, sliced

- 6 garlic cloves, smashed

- 2 whole star anise

- 1 cinnamon stick

- 1 Tbsp coriander seeds

- 1 Tbsp fennel seeds

- 1 Tbsp whole black peppercorns

- Optional fish sauce, mushrooms, greens and rice noodles

- Preheat oven to 425°F. Place bones on baking sheet and roast 20 minutes until browned.

- Transfer bones to large pot and add 8 cups water. Bring to boil then reduce heat to gently simmer 3 hours, skimming fat that rises to surface.

- Add onion, ginger, garlic and all spices. Simmer uncovered additional 3 hours.

- Turn off heat and allow broth to cool slightly before straining through fine mesh sieve. Discard solids.

- Optional to season broth with few tablespoons fish sauce.

- Transfer broth back to pot. Bring to gentle simmer and add varieties of sliced mushrooms, greens like bok choy and rice noodles. Cook an additional 5 minutes before serving.

Blueberry Cardamom Smoothie Bowl

- 2 cups frozen blueberries

- 1 large frozen banana

- 1 cup nut milk

- 1 Tbsp almond butter

- 1 tsp vanilla extract

- 1/2 tsp ground cardamom

- Topping Options: granola, shredded coconut, cacao nibs, goji berries, bee pollen, pumpkin seeds

- Add blueberries, banana, milk, almond butter, vanilla and cardamom to blender. Puree until thick smoothie consistency reached.

- Divide evenly between two bowls. Generously top with any combination of suggested toppings.

Black Bean Chocolate Cake

- 1 15-ounce can black beans, drained and rinsed

- 3 eggs

- 1/3 cup maple syrup

- 1/4 cup olive oil

- 1/4 cup unsweetened cacao powder

- 2 tsp baking powder

- 1 tsp vanilla

- 1/2 tsp salt

- Optional 1/2 cup chocolate chips

- Preheat oven to 350°F. Grease 8x8 inch baking pan.

- Combine all ingredients except chocolate chips in high powered blender. Puree until completely smooth batter formed.

- Fold in chocolate chips if using. Pour batter into prepared pan, smooth top gently.

- Bake 30-35 minutes until toothpick inserted in center comes out clean. Allow to cool slightly before cutting.

Overnight Pumpkin Spice Oats

- 1 cup steel cut oats

- 2 cups almond milk

- 1/4 cup canned pumpkin

- 1 Tbsp maple syrup

- 1 Tbsp chia seeds

- 2 tsp pumpkin pie spice

- 1 tsp vanilla extract

- 1 pinch salt

- Optional: nuts, seeds, nut butter, fruit to top

- Combine all ingredients except toppings in container with sealable lid. Mix thoroughly until fully incorporated.

- Seal and refrigerate overnight, at least 8 hours and up to 3 days.

- Remove from fridge in morning when ready to eat. Top with any combination of nuts, seeds, nut butter and fruit before enjoying. Consider pecans, sunflower seeds, almond butter, bananas or berries!

Carrot Salad Wraps

- 4 whole grain wraps or collard greens

- 2-3 carrots, shredded

- 1 cucumber, shredded

- 1 mango, cubed

- 1 avocado, cubed

- 1 cup mixed sprouts

- Tahini Maple Dressing:

- 1/4 cup tahini

- 2 Tbsp lemon juice

- 1 Tbsp maple syrup

- 1 garlic clove, minced

- 2 Tbsp water

- Pinch cayenne

- Whisk all dressing ingredients until smooth drizzle-able sauce texture forms. Set aside.

- Assemble wraps by evenly dividing shredded carrot, cucumber, mango, avocado and sprouts between tortillas or wide collard leaves.

- Drizzle desired amount of dressing over fillings.

- Tightly roll wraps up and slice diagonally if desired.

- Enjoy these veggie packed wraps with refreshing maple tahini dressing!

Immune Recovery Chicken Noodle Soup

- 1 pound chicken breasts or thighs

- 8 cups chicken broth

- 3 carrots, sliced

- 3 celery stalks, sliced

- 1 onion, diced

- 3 garlic cloves, minced

- 1 Tbsp fresh ginger, grated

- 2 Tbsp fresh thyme, chopped

- 1 bay leaf

- 8 ounces dry egg noodles

- 2 cups baby spinach

- 1/4 cup parsley, chopped

- Add chicken, broth, carrots, celery, onion, garlic, ginger, thyme and bay leaf to large pot. Bring to boil over medium high heat.

- Reduce heat to gently simmer for 15 minutes.

- Remove chicken and shred with two forks once cool enough to handle. Return shredded meat to soup pot.

- Raise heat again until broth boils. Add egg noodles and cook 8 minutes until just tender.

- Remove bay leaf. Add spinach and parsley, simmer 1 additional minute.

- Adjust seasoning as needed. Serve piping hot to nourish back to health!

Chapter 13: Transitioning to an Immune-Friendly Lifestyle

Implementing insight distilled from extensive nutritional science into workable habits with lasting compliance proves vital for successfully translating informed theory into measurable reality through sustained action. Beyond just possessing evidence-based knowledge, activating improved consequences depends on effectively adopting practices that encode desired principles into unconscious routine.

While the dilemma of disconnected information and behavior plagues many domains like fitness, finance and environmentalism, the divide particularly hinders healthcare. Though life-saving insights now demonstrate how adjusting eating patterns prevents and reverses chronic disease, actually adhering to ideal models for shopping, cooking and dining frequently stalls even among the well-educated and motivated.

If knowledgeable physicians fail converting medical knowledge into self-care compliance, how much prevention potential remains squandered for unsupported public groups attempting similar feats solo? Fortunately, research into lifestyle psychology uncovers several key insights that can bridge this persistent gap for establishing automated wellness habits with long-term adherence.

Find Supportive Community

Perhaps the most vital technique for sustaining motivation involves joining a supportive community pursuing similar growth. Humans evolved as deeply social creatures, forging purpose and identity through shared norms, beliefs and aspirations that facilitate group bonding. By harnessing this innate hunger to belong within circles resonating core values through accountability, inspiration, emotional validation and resource exchange, fledgling initiatives can crystallize into integral lifestyles.

Seeking like-minded members with overlapping interests provides a nurturing atmosphere that normalizes and reinforces desired habits through continual engagement, empathy, celebration of small wins, and constructive input around obstacles. Shared experience enriches wisdom.

Mastermind groups, MeetUp gatherings, family participation, book/cooking clubs or private social media groups all enable rewarding camaraderie that demystifies the path ahead, reminding individuals they do not walk alone when confronting deep change.

Start Slowly & Simply

Rather than extreme dietary overhauls prone to rapid failure through impractical intensity, adopt gradual continual enhancements through progressive layering aligned to intrinsic priorities. Sustainable change unfolds across unintimidating modifications that avoid reactionary rejection. Have patience.

Focus first solely on crowding out inflammatory refined oils or decreasing additive-laden processed items. As healthier substitutions normalize, purposefully augment produce variety, beans/lentils intake or ethical animal proteins as sensible next steps rather than demanding simultaneous perfection upfront.

Once modest beginnings root through this adjustable part-by-part segmented approach with flexible timelines, identity shifts naturally evolve perspectives that motivate maturing tastes toward more radical remodeling as evidence of benefits accumulate. But restraint early on gives space for self-acceptance to grow around changes.

Design Consistent Meal Templates

Consistent menus constructed around efficient batch cooking empowers sustainment by reducing daily decisions that risk fluctuating motivation. Structure powerfully supports habit formation through stable rhythm.

Reliable recipes prepared weekly in bulk with simple additions like sauteed greens or crisp salads minimize meal redundancy while granting effortless nutrition. Ongoing spoon-fed creativity reignites passion lost steaming repetitive chicken and broccoli.

For time-restricted individuals, guide regular weekly planning using certain dishes as staple meal foundations allowing adjustable sides. Depending on lifestyle factors, this may include a rotating set of staples like cooked grains, prepped proteins, marinated vegetables, hearty soups and loose recipes to splice into quick combinations as needed.

Bridge Habits To Existing Rituals

Rather than imposing wholly foreign behaviors, adaptively infiltrate evidence-based activities into current normalized routines for minimizing friction through tapping existing unconscious patterns. This integration approach improves compliance through minimal disruption felt by those affected who implicitly welcome the intentions already.

For example, augmenting established morning smoothies with anti-inflammatory turmeric or a daily multivitamin merges into natural flow easier than forcing alien practices like intermittent fasting upon resistant minds holding longtime breakfast attachment. Meet people within established ritual before reshaping entirely.

Latch new actions onto old habitual triggers by creatively substituting components once pattern activation occurs. This inside reform continues identity traditions valued across generations while gently improving consequences through incremental steps centered on inheritance.

Make It Easy To Remember

Despite sincere aspirations for elevating wellness, the demands of hurried modernity often relegate even important intentions like taking supplements or special meal prep to background noise as focus fixates on urgent deadlines, family obligations or pending crises.

By externally encoding behavioral prompts into unconscious environs, decisions transition from unreliable disciplined effort to automatic contextual response. Visual checklists, scheduler alerts, preparatory trigger locations, packaged pre-made items and reminder notes dissolve need for active remembering already strained.

This tangible environmental integration weaves intended actions into existing flow rather than battling limited cognitive bandwidth with unsustainable white-knuckle determination alone. Maps make foreign terrain familiar enough to navigate comfortably. External structures sustain progress when distraction inevitably overwhelms conscious resolve.

Disarm Stress Before It Disables Progress

Finally, appreciating the unavoidable reality of recurring external stress that sabotages resolve honors human fallibility while erasing self-judgment that worsens outcomes. By proactively accepting periodic deviation when turbulent events trigger instinctive coping relief, readiness to resume course restores faster without toxic shame that promotes relapse.

Allow occasional intentional indulgence to discharge pent up deprivation before it erupts into binge through restrained denial. Neutralize guilt's self-amplifying power by intentionally planning strategic timed exception windows beforehand as a pressure release valve for reliable resuming.

An 80/20 lifestyle diet approach accepts imperfect consistency across days by consciously designing rewarding target ratios that expect periodic exemption. This self-compassion retains positive progress momentum in the same direction rather than hijacking sustainable advancement through rigid absolutism doomed for distress-driven failure.

Through communal encouragement, gradualist steps, steady environment, rhythmic rituals and stress-preempting leniency that compassionately coaxes incremental improvement, aspiring intentions crystallize into automatic lifestyle habits that feel effortless through phases of conscious incompetence to unconscious competence. Lasting transformation unfolds through progressive self-discovery, not instant perfection.

Part IV: Beyond Diet - Supporting Immune Resilience

With extensive ground now covered exploring evidence-based dietary selections to fuel intricate molecular machinery governing human immune response, additional lifestyle factors beyond food alone profoundly impact holistic disease resilience as well.

While essential nutrients provide raw construction materials for fabricating protective proteins and signaling compounds, optimal functional infrastructure depends greatly upon physiological environments suitably primed through stress-minimizing behaviors and routines that enable restorative rest.

By supporting healthy function of detoxification organs, nervous tone regulation, circadian biology and psychiatric balance through certain non-dietary practices, profound benefit synergistically amplifies nutrition's immune-supporting potential.

Fortunately, ancient sciences of traditional healing systems emphasize connecting nutrition with broader preventative rituals for harmonizing the mind-body ecosystem - combining medicinal fare with balancing movement routines, community wellness practices, mental hygiene through meditation and adequate sleep.

Modern science now illuminates these effective pairings further, revealing specific biomechanisms like cortisol's immunosuppression and melatonin's anticancer activity that mechanistically detail traditional wisdom on healing lifestyles beyond just eating herbs alone.

While by no means exhaustive, Part IV explores integrating supplemental areas impacting disease susceptibility that interdependently regulate core physiology alongside diet - the orchestrating conductor that directs material conversion into somatic function. Embrace nutrition as centerpiece amidst larger lifestyle mosaic where non-food components prove equally essential to flourishing.

Now that previous sections built strong conceptual foundation detailing interconnections between diverse molecular immune pathways and how functional foods feed these systems, we widen lenses to appreciate external terrain-shaping influences that determine phenotypic expression potentials from underlying genotype.

This socio-environmental dimension proves critical, as certain individuals despite making all evidence-backed dietary improvements still battle conditions from past or present stress, trauma, toxicity, disrupted circadian signaling, microbiome imbalance and other engrained factors scrambling systemic homeostasis. Without addressing these root sources destabilizing intrinsic physiology, even ideal nutrition insufficiently breaches boundaries separating knowledge and lasting positive transformation.

Fortunately supporting healthy regulation of stress reactivity, sleep hygiene, toxin elimination and microbiome commensals through holistic healing modalities synergizes numerous lifestyle components into powerful delivery vectors that infuse nutrition's immune benefits deep into human experience - bridging intellectual grokking to embodied genomic manifestation. Let vitality flourish

through cooperative lifestyle cultivation paired with proper
fuel.

Chapter 14: Managing Stress for Immune Health

Beyond assailing pathogens, the elaborate architecture of human immunity equally battles disruptive stress that perpetuates fight-or-flight neural signaling maladapted for nuanced civilized life yet remains locked by primitive neurochemistry forged in brutish eras.

While brief arousal once focused faculties on life-saving response, unrelenting cortisol and catecholamine cascades now linked to systemic inflammation sabotage cellular repair and protective renewal necessary for maintaining resilient homeostasis across the lifespan.

By exploring lifestyle remedies that mitigate excessive sympathetic tone and hypothalamic-pituitary-adrenal (HPA) axis activation, proactive stress relief harmonizes holistic wellbeing centered on salutogenic neuroendocrine regulation - providing a balanced canvas for immunity to thrive within.

Stress & Immunity - Inescapable Impact

As introduced earlier, intrinsic survival responses rapidly unleashed in acutely dangerous contexts served vital purposes on hostile savannas yet prove wholly maladaptive for diffuse digital age anxieties that require more precise biochemistry supporting nuanced social cognition.

Unfortunately persistent perceived threats, uncertainty or conflict encoded within nervous circuitry locks physiology into an injury and starvation mindset that impairs higher faculties required for thriving modern demands. These reactively depressed capacities then feedback causing more environment mismatch, stress and helplessness.

Cortisol release blocks inflammation acutely yet becomes immunosuppressive longer term by blunting frontline lymphocytes and counterregulatory hormones that normally conclude sustained alarm. Anxiety-fueled adrenaline spikes glycate receptor proteins AGEing poor cell communication. Modern healthcare clearly overlooks root drivers for many downstream conditions.

Fortunately evidence-based holistic modalities now exist that ameliorate these destructive cycles earlier through nervous system relaxation, subconscious resolution, lifestyle balancing and community support - rather than symptomatic suppression after deep patterns manifest disease.

Restorative Movement Anchors Presence

bundle quick tension release practices into daily routines provide accessible portals for rapidly recentering physiology when unproductive reactions inevitably surface during ordinary challenges. Rather than requiring formal meditation or self-inquiry rigor, simple postural resets gently calm fight/flight axis activation while enhancing mindfulness of stuck mental/physical patterns that limit conscious choice.

For example briefly walking barefoot outdoors connecting sensory experience to surroundings dissolves distraction while lowering cortisol, inflammation and anxiety consequently. Gentle neck stretches with slow nasal breathing similarly defuses repetitive thinking by opening airways for oxygenating circulation to settle regions flooded with stress chemicals.

Even basic shoulder rolls, toe wiggles or hip circles inject casual relief into long days before emotional triggers hijack higher logic and cellular repair operations. By thoughtfully scattering these minute nervous system relaxation touchpoints across fixed schedules, considerable compound alleviation manifests organically without demanding profound ritual transformation initially. Incorporate as reminders arise.

Community Aligns Values with Lifestyle

Beyond transient practices like stretches or breathing that provide temporary yet vital nervous stabilization, establishing regular social gatherings for sharing communal support, resources and perspectives allows individuals to step out of isolated psychological patterns into inspiring spaces that align values with lifestyles for sustaining motivation.

Group dialogue grounds lofty theories around ideal wellness into practical neighborhood contexts of cooking, childcare, financial limitations, career pressures and relational anxieties that often overwhelm isolated good intentions. By voices airing candid concerns without judgment and finding empathy from those overcoming similar struggles, motivation crystallizes through feeling understood while also being reminded of purpose. The lone mountain climb seems impossible without a guiding team.

Ongoing community wellness meetups offer replenishing fuel for continually advancing health goals through reciprocal nurturing care that our alienated modern society largely lacks. Shared experience builds momentum.

Reframing Stress as Exciting Challenge

Yet even amidst supportive circles, the subjective nature of perceived stress leaves experiential existence subject to cognitive interpretation. By reframing bodily arousal as excitement rather than anxiety, racing heartbeats and sweaty palms become framed as natural responses anticipating resolve and growth rather than debilitating distress.

Simple conscious reattribution without changing actual circumstance dramatically empowers students before intimidating exams, athletes before competition, and employees before critical presentations to channel that mobilized vigor as focused motivation to overcome difficulty through reappraisal of narrative context around what sensations imply.

This intrinsic leadership direction of assigning meaning amidst adversity trains mastery over environmental factors that otherwise trigger panic by routing physiology through opportunistic value rather than victimized threat when faced with the unknown. Stress becomes subjective ally, not incapacitating foe.

Overall by implementing lifestyle practices that regulation baseline nervous tone, befriending healthy community support and reframing arousal as affirming adventures, the inevitable uncertainty around work, health and relationships transforms from source of despair to growth adventures required for actualizing full human potential. Our perception crafts cellular reality.

Chapter 15: The Importance of Sleep

Beyond dietary choices, few lifestyle factors more profoundly support or suppress immune system functioning than quality and quantity of nightly sleep. Far more than just stole downtime, recent discoveries reveal intricate biological processes activating each night during sleep cycles that effectively direct nocturnal cleaning and repair operations across tissues - clearing molecular debris while optimizing cells for next day activity demands.

Failing to prioritize adequate sleep durably sabotages this indispensable night shift biological work crew attempting vital custodial tasks - allowing dysfunctional structures and inflammatory signals to gradually accumulate, eventually hindering routine physiology. Fortunately, studies confirm simple consistent sleep hygiene measures that enhance this innate self-recovery capacity, thereby bolstering longevity and disease resilience over time.

Sleep Regulates Immune Crosstalk

Two way communication exists where the sleep-wake cycle heavily influences immune activity while specific immune chemicals signal the brain, shaping sleep architecture quality based on current physiological status.

The cytokine IL-1 notably builds each night as incomplete daily tasks tag cellular trash for overnight lysosomal and proteasomal activity. If excess accrues from chronic stress or disease, escalated IL-1 levels interfere with restorative slow wave and REM sleep. This catch-22 limits needed recovery.

Likewise melatonin production from natural light/dark patterns helps activate nocturnal macrophage activity against bacterial invaders through receptor binding, whereas sleep deprivation conversely impairs natural killer cell ADCC tumor toxicity and neutrophil bacterial phagocytosis.

Optimized sleep clearly coordinates mutually beneficial immune regulation through bidirectional chemical signaling feedback loops that select immune responses and intensities based on homeostatic requirements across 24 hour solar cycles.

Infection Risk Increases Without Sleep

Both animal models and human studies consistently demonstrate increased infection susceptibility from insufficient sleep due to broad immune disturbance including natural killer cell loss, decreased T cell activation, reduced IgA salivary antibodies and subdued signaling to bolster adaptive responses.

Models of bacterial infection after just 24 hours sleep deprivation show markedly reduced pulmonary macrophage and lymphocyte recruitment to lung tissue along with 2-3 times higher pathogen quantities from suppressed immune reactions - allowing infections to swiftly strengthen once resilience deficits compound without reset.

Similar elevated viral infection rates follow sleep-restricted individuals with hydrocortisone studies showing glucocorticoids temporarilyRequested exert comparable immune impairment. Simply allowing adequate restorative sleep appropriately calibrates needed immunity against opportunistic threats whereas chronic sleep disruption leaves us vulnerable just as concerning modern lifestyle epidemics spread globally.

Sleep Clears Molecular Waste

Until recently, the observable suspended neural activity and slowed metabolism during sleep fostered notions of a dormant state with assumed declining importance relative youth. However exponential discovery reveals sleep instead directs profound physiological renewal unachievable during waking hours alone.

Deeper NREM slow wave sleep (SWS) effectively triggers cellular cleaning operations through amplified cerebrospinal ATP-driven efflux pumping lymph channels that double extracellular fluid (ECF) volume, creating needed space for diffusive soluble proteins to migrate out from congested intracellular zones.

This osmotic gradient allows waste removal during sustained neural inactivity without interference for trafficking essential nutrients like glucose and oxygen normally required awake. Support cells further shrink during SWS, expanding ECF channels for heightened paravascular clearance of amyloids and other neurotoxic byproducts that impair next day plasticity if uncleared.

Growth and psychic health depend deeply on sufficient sleep.

Sleep Supports DNA Repair

Alongside clearing proteinaceous waste through lymphatic and glial activity each night, sleep also supports critical DNA repair duties necessary for healthy cell replication and hazard resilience long term.

Nucleotides face constant damage threats from metabolism byproducts like reactive oxygen species along with radiation exposure and chemical genotoxins requiring continual mending to uphold genetic integrity stabilizing life.

While nuclear and mitochondrial genomes utilize elaborate molecular editing systems during daytime activity, highest DNA repair activity occurs during nightly sleep cycles through selection of priority injury sites based on transcriptional relevance.

About 90% DNA repair processes transpire during sleep, ensuring homeostatic renewal against perpetual decay dynamics. Even modest nightly shortfalls sabotage this essential maintenance for withstanding modern molecular instability. Prioritizing sleep pays exponential dividends over lifespan.

Tips For Improving Sleep Hygiene

Though one third of life drifts away through fleeting rest, society still broadly disregards sleep health to its own systemic detriment. Disrupted circadian biology from insufficient or inconsistent sleep chronically activates fight flight responses with sympathetic hyperarousal conversely impairing parasympathetic Rest & Digest relaxation. This precludes cellular rejuvenation from sleep deprivation.

By incorporating more of the following beneficial practices, internal homeostatic renewal operated through programmed sleep again flourishes:

- **Develop consistent bed & wake times** even across weekends to reinforce circadian signals through reliability.

- **Avoid bright light after dusk** letting melatonin naturally rise while limiting electronics/screens that suppress endogenous secretions.

- **Cut caffeine after noon, alcohol before bed** as both disrupt sleep architecture and impede deeper dream states.

- **Create total darkness** through blackout curtains with cooler bedroom temperatures around 65 degrees Fahrenheit.

- **Establish relaxing pre-bed rituals** like journaling, tea sipping, meditating, gentle yoga or reading fiction to ease the mind downshifting into sleep.

- **Consider earplugs and eye masks** if needed to reduce sensory disruptions for those more sensitive maintaining REM cycles.

- **Try to sleep when sleepy, awaken when alert** - following intrinsic chronorhythms tied to sun cycles.

- **Limit large meals before bed** to allow digestive processes to wane while enabling deeper parasympathetic relaxation.

As the most nourishing activity we engage each day, responsibly satisfying sleep frees profound regenerative biological processes to uphold systemic functioning across years. Dreams retune neural pathways for next day tissue restoration. Prioritize rest nightly for lifelong immunological resilience!

Conclusion: A Lifetime of Robust Immunity

We arrive at the concluding passage fortified through exploration of diverse scientific insights and cultural wisdom that collectively uphold immune health as the dynamic interdependent culmination of lifestyle behaviors balancing myriad processes governing lifelong holistic wellbeing.

From this synthesized perspective that embraces physiology as an elegantly unified whole, targeted pharmaceuticals that haphazardly dictate isolated biochemical pathways inevitably lose efficacy over a lifetime. Whereas informed nutrition and lifestyle adjustments cooperating with innate biology proves sustainably capable of gently upholding daily function against disorder through perpetual nourishment of interconnected systems.

By responsibly applying evidence-based daily practices cultivated through ancestral logic onto modern living environments, the immune system persists exquisitely capable of upholding vigilant defenses through nourishment of progenitor cells towards continual measured renewal against unremitting entropy dynamics across decades of use.

Immunity as Systemic Equilibrium

With deeper revelation of immune physiology as a profoundly harmonized network that skillfully maintains equilibrium signaling between varied tissues through nutritional bioactives, beneficial microbes, homeostatic hormones and balanced nerve conduits, notions of simply forcing higher qualitative metrics like antibody counts or inflammatory biomarkers no longer maintains logical sense.

Effective immune vigor relies on delicate equilibrium kinetics between activation pathways and resolute counter-regulators that selectively check only unnecessary excessive responses while retaining poised defensiveness against opportunistic threats. Blindly pushing isolated arms of this elegant system inevitably yields adverse outcomes over time.

Strengthening particular muscle groups through focused exercise rightly increases their stunted performance contributing to whole body coordination. Whereas the fibroblast cells generating collagenous connective tissues linking interdependent muscle, nerve and vascular networks warrant equal nourishing care for delivering their role upholding systematic integrity from which all power flows during exertion.

With connective health intact, focused training logically bolsters athleticism. But without balanced nourishment upholding systemic integration from cellular to holistic ranks, isolated gains prove transient as foundational support falters. The human immune system operates by the same irrefutable principles.

Transition From Avoiding Pathology to Nourishing Potential

This revelations warrants marked transition in health strategy - from primitive destructive "attack and kill" mentalities against invading pathogens towards cultivation of sustainable daily practices that nourish the fertile soil upholding those formidable layered defenses through perpetual renewal against unrelenting modern dysbiotic pressures.

Rather than destroying disease and rushing to return to former codependent lifestyles that inevitably enabled those opportunistic breakdowns in the first place, discovery of our own true healing potential heralds conscious departure from former programming towards courageous self-actualization.

Radical lifestyle rebirth often holds far greater promise than brief symptomatic respite before recrudescent pathology reemerges downstream from sustained causal factors of ignorance and neglect. With open eyes and bold hearts we walk gently into the good night having nourished our deepest intrinsic capacity for self-healing using ample wisdom passed down through generations.

Commit To Continual Growth Through Daily Practice

Transitioning from passive pill popping patient awaiting sickness towards proactive cultivation of lifelong radical wellness through perpetual practice requires commitment to incremental progressional improvements through stages of mastery.

Spectacular instant gratification promises unfortunately rarely deliver sustainable solutions to crept systemic dysfunction decades in the making. However leaning into realistic routine small steps forwards ultimately traverses vast distances over years. With consistent gentle nourishment, dormant human potential stirs guiding us home.

From that empowered state of perpetual development we refrain from judging others still embarking on their early passages - for we too once maintained similar limitations requiring compassionate guidance from those further along uplifting behind them. And with boundless opportunity always awaiting activation of insight, even the wise remain perpetually students to the emerging futures our boldest dreams might yet manifest.

On this never ending co-creative journey thriving inside uncertainty through mystery and wonder, remember to celebrate small daily victories of nourishment against entropy because cumulatively those individual incremental improvements pave the certain path towards sustained systemic health-span through our deepest healing potential.

Just as immune health relies on balanced equilibrium homeostasis across years, so too should your lifestyle practices seek sustainable gains by cooperating with biology for the long play rather than forcing transitory change through rigid ascetic denial of intrinsic human needs ultimately requiring some measured indulgence.

With ample science-supported understanding now cultivated towards immune competence and the many interconnected pillars upholding such vast nuanced networks through dietary nourishment of microbiome communities, detoxification pathways, metabolic flexibility, psychoemotional stress resilience and adequate restorative sleep, you hold sufficient knowledge needed to feed formidable lifelong defenses.

Now go play, go create and boldly walk the path of courage strengthened through daily practices advancing radical whole-body wellness! With consistent mindfulness towards maintaining homeostatic equilibrium across interconnected lifestyle behaviors, robust immunity persists eminently within reach.

About the Author

As a naturopathic physician, I'm driven each day by inspiration gleaned through witnessing the incredible human capacity for holistic healing once simple nourishment is provided. After years consulting clients on personalized nutrition plans, I felt urged to compile my insights distilling core dietary wisdom supporting foundational wellbeing.

Far beyond chasing miracles obsessing over exotic superfood fads, authentic health means embracing traditional whole food preparations that synergistically nourish a spectrum of interconnected physiological processes regulating resilience against modern pressures. I'm humbled receiving vulnerably candid stories of positive life transformations achieved through basic lifestyle adjustments guided by this compassionate integrative approach.

While formal medical degrees and curated knowledge rightfully signify certain mastery, nothing replaces direct empathetic understanding of suffering acquired sitting with people through their darkest moments of doubt on paths towards reclaimed wellness. My intermittent fasting journey through an autoimmune diagnosis gave me priceless firsthand experience that perpetual uncertainty poses the greatest challenge behind sustainable behavior change.

Through turbulent phases of growth, I've learned self-acceptance and loving community foster empowered self-care. Now thriving beyond former limitations, I feel blessed paying forward the grace I've received by striving to intuitively meet people wherever they stand today with empathy, hoping thoughtful evidence-based suggestions may inspire your enriched tomorrows beyond wildest imagination. Just know, you've already begun the heroic emergence. Keep going...

www.ingramcontent.com/pod-product-compliance
Lightning Source LLC
Chambersburg PA
CBHW070858260726
48661CB00004B/1477